"In these times, where queer and trans people are continually the targets of violence, discrimination, and archaic public accommodation policies, it is hopeful and necessary that we focus on power and resilience. *The Queer and Transgender Resilience Workbook* is a useful and refreshing guide to the possibilities of restoration and transformation for queer and transgender people."

> —**Holiday Simmons, MSW**, social justice advocate, facilitator, public speaker, and healer

"We each have an opportunity to explore ourselves profoundly as we evolve in our lives as queer and trans people, and this workbook provides unique and engaging guidance. Enjoy exploring your resilient self!"

> —**Danielle Castro, MA, MFT**, director of research for the Center of Excellence for Transgender Health at the University of California, San Francisco

T0301075

THE
QUEER &
TRANSGENDER
RESILIENCE
WORKBOOK

Skills for Navigating Sexual Orientation & Gender Expression

ANNELIESE SINGH, PhD, LPC

NEW HARBINGER PUBLICATIONS, INC.

Publisher's Note

This publication is designed to provide accurate and authoritative information in regard to the subject matter covered. It is sold with the understanding that the publisher is not engaged in rendering psychological, financial, legal, or other professional services. If expert assistance or counseling is needed, the services of a competent professional should be sought.

NEW HARBINGER PUBLICATIONS is a registered trademark of New Harbinger Publications, Inc.

New Harbinger Publications is an employee-owned company.

Distributed in Canada by Raincoast Books

Copyright © 2018 by Anneliese A. Singh
New Harbinger Publications, Inc.
5720 Shattuck Avenue
Oakland, CA 94609
www.newharbinger.com

Cover design by Amy Shoup

Acquired by Ryan Buresh

Edited by Kristi Hein

All Rights Reserved

Library of Congress Cataloging-in-Publication Data

Names: Singh, Anneliese A., author.

Title: The queer and transgender resilience workbook : skills for navigating sexual orientation and gender expression / Anneliese Singh, PhD, LPC.

Description: Oakland, CA : New Harbinger Publications, Inc., [2018] | Includes bibliographical references.

Identifiers: LCCN 2017058868 (print) | LCCN 2017060685 (ebook) | ISBN 9781626259478 (PDF e-book) | ISBN 9781626259485 (ePub) | ISBN 9781626259461 (pbk. : alk. paper)

Subjects: LCSH: Gays--Identity. | Transgender people--Identity. | Resilience (Personality trait) | Self-esteem. | Sexual orientation. | Gender nonconformity.

Classification: LCC HQ76.25 (ebook) | LCC HQ76.25 .S566 2018 (print) | DDC 306.76--dc23

LC record available at https://lccn.loc.gov/2017058868

Printed in the United States of America

26   25   24

10   9   8   7

For Lenny Zenith, Jeanine Grimes, Cherie Schwab, the city of New Orleans, and the country of India—you all taught me everything I needed to know about being resilient and embracing the queer and trans parts of me I was taught by society to hide.

For my beloved, Lauren Lukkarila—each step with you is a sacred unfolding that not only makes me a better person but also helps me be more of who I truly am. I love you with all of me!

For the queer and trans community of Atlanta—may we all continue to manifest the liberation movements rooted in beloved community, equity, and justice.

For all the queer and trans liberation movements around the world—our lives and histories are ancient and beautiful. May we remember our true and deepest liberation within ourselves, and with one another, more and more.

Contents

Foreword
by Diane Ehrensaft

It is afternoon, June 23, 2017. With great pleasure, I am sitting at my computer in Oakland, California, writing the foreword to *The Queer and Trans Resilience Workbook*. This day also marks the start of the 45th annual San Francisco Pride celebration, opening with the Trans March later today. And what is the theme of this year's Trans March? "Celebrating Resilience with Love and Resistance"—a title chosen, I'm speculating, without ever having seen Anneliese Singh's inspiring workbook, given that it is not yet in print. My point: resilience is in the air, having been discovered by so many of us as the crux of health, well-being, and transcendence for the LGBTQ community. For so many years, in trying to make a more equitable and accepting world, we have focused on teaching tolerance. Now it is time to teach resilience—the inner strength and centered sense of self and community that is never a given but rather a communal accomplishment.

Allow me to go back in time for a moment. First let me situate myself. I am a cisgender straight woman, pronouns she/her/hers, a dyed-in-the-wool feminist of the 1960s, a mother of a grown-up gay son (once a gender expansive little boy), and the director of mental health of the Child and Adolescent Gender Center. So now let's visit 1967. I was a senior in college and graduating from the honors psych program at University of Michigan. Our faculty advisor called a meeting of all the women in the program. He sat us all down and advised us not to apply to graduate school because we would only take up men's spaces and later drop out to get married and have babies. He showed us a graph of dropout rates of female compared to male graduate students to prove his point. We were stunned, but not one of us stormed out or stormed at him in the face of his egregious sexist macroaggression. Instead, our revenge was to go on to get PhDs—every single one of us. In a way, we exercised our resilience through action, but not in a way that would stop that same faculty advisor from delivering the same outrageous message to the next cohort of women in the honors psych program. If only we'd had resilience building similar to what Singh so expertly offers to the LGBTQ community in the workbook you are about to embark on, it could have been better.

LGBTQ resilience—what's it all about? It's about coming out to yourself and then coming out to others, on your own timeline. It's about recognizing the evolution of gender and sexuality across your lifetime—who you are today may change over time, and that's something to stand up for. It's about finding a positive mirror and using it—a reflection, from allies and loved ones, that who you are is authentic, expansive, and to be celebrated, rather than wrong, diminished, and to be rejected. It's about being mindful of the intersectionality in people's lives and making sure that we don't repeat experiences like what Anneliese Singh reported from her own childhood: "As a South Asian, multiracial, Sikh, queer, genderqueer femme…I struggled with my own resilience growing up. Messages abounded that there was something wrong with me, or that I didn't fit in—and unfortunately, there was no one around to tell me those things were not true and that my resilience to these experiences was important." It's about recognizing that if someone wants to know your gender or sexuality, it is not for them to say but for you to tell, or choose not to tell.

As you progress through the workbook, you will discover the important difference between homophobia and heterosexism, between transphobia and transnegativity, and between phobias, which are based on fear, and the "-ivities" and "-isms" that reflect bad actions. Building resilience requires boots on the ground to confront the bad actions that happen in everyday life. Ideally, breakdown of the phobias will organically follow.

I was trained psychoanalytically, and one of the biggest takeaways was that we all have conscious and unconscious layers, especially when it comes to gender and sexuality. It is no secret that psychoanalysis has not always been a friend to the LGBTQ community, but we can use the tools to our own benefit. Anneliese Singh implicitly does, seamlessly using the workbook to bring the unconscious to the light of day so it can be reworked into a more positive and empowered sense of self. It doesn't take being psychoanalyzed; rather, it takes setting aside time for reflection, metabolizing, and transcending. And that is building resilience.

To strengthen resilience is to enhance your own sense of agency. To fuel that sense of agency is to hope—to hope for yourself, to hope for a better future for everyone. As the workbook guides us to realize, it takes a village—yourself, your intimate others, the larger group around you. It is no longer Dale Evans crooning, "Have faith, hope, and charity, that's the way to live successfully" asking, "How do I know?" in her 1950s hit song, "The Bible Tells Me So." Now it's agency, hope, and resilience—and how do we know? Our LGBTQ community tells us so.

In my own work with gender diverse children and their families, I have conjured up the concepts of gender angels and gender ghosts. Gender angels are the internal messages that allow us to accept, support, and facilitate the growth of our youth in all their rainbows of gender iterations. Gender ghosts are the inner voices that whisper bad messages about people who dare to transgress gender norms or seem gender "different." Our task: to identify those messages and voices and promote victory of our gender angels over our gender ghosts. With *The Queer and Trans Resilience Workbook*, Anneliese Singh steps in to show us how to do this, not only with gender, but also with every facet of LGBTQ angels and ghosts. Just by holding this workbook in your hands you are already taking a big step toward shooing away the ghosts to make room for the angels. Now it is time to grab your pen and get to work.

Introduction
Why Resilience Is Important
for Queer and Trans People

This book is all about how you can be resilient, grow, and thrive if you are queer and trans. Whether you are just getting to know who you are as an LGBTQ (lesbian, gay, bisexual, trans, queer) person or whether you have been out to yourself and others for a long time—or somewhere in the middle—this book is designed to help you explore different aspects of who you are and what is important to you. Because queer and trans people can experience a range of stress, from stereotypes and misunderstandings to hate crimes and violence, it is critical that they understand resilience. In this book, I use "queer," "trans," and "LGBTQ" interchangeably as umbrella terms to capture those of us who are in the lesbian, gay, bisexual, trans, queer community. And, as I will discuss in Chapter 1, these terms can be woefully inadequate—and can also evolve pretty rapidly. So as you read this book, make sure you think and use the words that best describe *your* gender and sexual orientation identities.

What Is Resilience?

So, if resilience is so important, what is it? Resilience has been called the "ordinary magic" that you can use to bounce back from hard times (Masten, 2015). The best thing about resilience is that when you know how to tap into it, you can have an unlimited supply to draw from to navigate everyday challenges. Think of your own resilience as:

- Natural

- Something you can develop

- A set of skills you use to cope with adversity

- Developed intrapersonally (within you) and interpersonally (with others)

- Composed of strategies and processes over time

- Multiplied, the more you develop it

- Connected to thriving in the future

Over a decade of research has talked about the range of "minority stress" that queer and trans people experience—from being called names or feeling like you don't fit in to being kicked out of your home or being fired from a job (Meyer, 2003; 2015). This type of stress is incremental and insidious, adding up over time. When unchecked, minority stress can lead to hiding who you are and anticipating that others will hurt or judge you in some way. Even worse, you can internalize experiences of LGBTQ discrimination and anti-LGBTQ social messages, tricking you into believing that you are less worthy or valuable than straight and cisgender people.

Resilience helps you cope through stressful times, which is why resilience is so important. When you challenge internalized negative messages about being LGBTQ, embrace who you are, and remove obstacles from your life, your resilience multiplies and can help you live a more fulfilling and meaningful life. This book draws from resilience research with queer and trans people, making this information accessible and practical to apply in your daily life. It is full of activities—called *resilience practices*—that you can use to explore the unique resilience you have related to your gender and sexual orientation identities, as well as how to navigate life when faced with discrimination.

Opportunities to Grow Resilience

Because resilience is really a collection of coping strategies, you can think of acquiring resilience as a process, not just a onetime event. Let's say you hear someone call you a bad name or make fun of you for being queer or trans. The first time, you may be so shocked you don't say anything. You go home and replay the event over and over in your mind, wishing you had said something. This is not quite resilience. Rather, you risk beating yourself up and internalizing shame for other people's discriminatory acts.

Let's say the next time something like this occurs, you talk it over with an LGBTQ ally—someone who really supports you as an LGBTQ person—and you both role-play ways you can hold on to your self-worth in these types of situations. Bingo! That is resilience. As a result, the next time you hear that same person or someone else say anti-LGBTQ things to you, you do something different—like feeling proud of your LGBTQ identity and standing up for yourself. Double bingo! That is all resilience too.

So resilience can involve the things you feel and do as an individual to take care of yourself (*intrapersonal* resilience) when bad things happen, and it can involve reaching out to supportive people as sources of strength (*interpersonal* resilience). Resilience develops over time, so you have many opportunities to develop resilience. You can think about resilience as the intrapersonal and interpersonal sources of strength you can draw on to get through those tough times and adapt to change. There is also the resilience you can develop from being part of a collective group who share identities, values, or some other commonality (*community* resilience), such as being part of a community of trans people of color. The greater your awareness of these sources, the more readily you can remember to use them to bounce back to your regular self.

Resilience Strategies and Skills for Queer and Trans People

Just as I am using "queer," "trans," and "LGBTQ" as umbrella terms for many identities that potentially fall somewhere within them, you can think about resilience as an umbrella term as well for the toolbox of knowledge and strategies crucial to helping you get through hard times as a queer or trans person. In this book, I discuss ten resilience strategies you can develop and grow to increase your overall resilience and well-being. At the core of your own resilience as an LGBTQ person is your ability to define your gender identity and sexual orientation for yourself. I talk about this core resilience strategy in Chapter 1 (*Getting Real: Defining Your LGBTQ Self in a World That Demands Conformity*). In subsequent chapters, you learn how to develop the ten components of this core resilience:

- *You Are More Than Your Gender and Sexual Orientation* (Chapter 2)—Learn to identify what other identities shape your resilience as queer or trans.

- *Further Identifying Negative Messages* (Chapter 3)—Pinpoint the specific messages you have learned about your sexual orientation, gender, and other important identities (such as race/ethnicity, social class, disability).

- *Knowing Your Self-Worth* (Chapter 4)—Identify how to learn your self-worth and grow your self-esteem.

- *Standing Up for Yourself* (Chapter 5)—Learn how to speak up for yourself as an LGBTQ person.

- *Affirming and Enjoying Your Body* (Chapter 6)—Explore how you feel about your body and how to affirm your physical self.

- *Building Relationships and Creating Community* (Chapter 7)—Develop skills in standing up for yourself and being assertive.

- *Getting Support and Knowing Your Resources* (Chapter 8)—Learn what helps you be resilient and how to get your needs met.

- *Getting Inspired* (Chapter 9)—Reflect on how feeling hopeful can grow resilience and how to be inspired and learn new and different things about yourself.

- *Making Change and Giving Back* (Chapter 10)—Think about how your resilience is related to helping others and getting involved in positive social change.

- *Growing and Thriving* (Chapter 11)—Set resilience goals for practicing self-love, self-growth, and self-reflection to thrive in your life as an LGBTQ person.

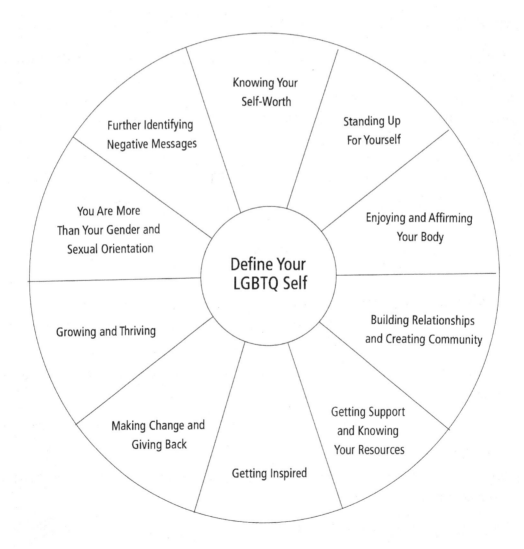

These eleven resilience strategies build upon one another and multiply the more you develop them. The Queer and Trans Resilience Wheel encompasses the dynamic and evolving nature of these resilience strategies. The core resilience in the wheel is how you define your own LGBTQ self. The starting and ending points of the resilience wheel are flexible: you can jump to any "spoke" at any point and work to further develop that element of your resilience.

Each chapter in this book corresponds to one of these spokes, exploring that resilience strategy in more depth. Therefore, as you move through each chapter, you are developing a facet of your resilience as described on a spoke of the resilience wheel, building on your previous learning and strengthening your overall resilience.

With each chapter's resilience practices you can explore and assess your current levels of resilience in order to identify next steps you want to take to grow your resilience as an LGBTQ person. I encourage you to be as real with yourself as possible in these resilience practices, because these practices are designed specifically for your own exploration. You are worth it! You may choose to share some of what you are learning about yourself and your resilience as you go (like with a supportive friend, family member, or counselor), but the choice is yours. As you get to the end of each chapter, a resilience wrap-up summarizes the chapter's major learning points related to your resilience. It is a time to pause and review your learning. You can also return to read these sections if you decide to go back and review a certain aspect of resilience.

I wrote this workbook because I have spent the last two decades researching queer and trans resilience. As a South Asian, multiracial, Sikh, queer, genderqueer femme (I will talk about some of these words in the next few chapters), I struggled with my own resilience as I was growing up. Messages abounded that there was something wrong with me, or that I didn't fit in—and unfortunately, there was no one around to tell me those things were not true and that my resilience to these experiences was important. I wrote this workbook because, whether through my research findings or by learning things in my personal life, I have found a big bonus in becoming more resilient to discrimination: the more you believe in your value as an LGBTQ person, the more empowered and happy you become! And that is what the world actually needs more of—more happy, empowered, liberated, and affirmed queer and trans people who know they are valuable and loved and are treated with respect and dignity. You are an important part of that world! So now let's get started, in Chapter 1, exploring your resilience related to your own sexual orientation and gender identities.

Getting Real
Defining Your LGBTQ Self in a World That Demands Conformity

This chapter is an opportunity to take some time to reflect on how much you have learned about being queer and trans from other people, and then sifting through some of those messages to learn more about your own gender and sexual orientation identities. Research suggests that a large part of queer and trans resilience boils down to being able to define these identities for yourself (Singh, Hays, & Watson, 2011; Singh & McKleroy, 2011; Singh, Meng, & Hansen, 2014). Let's explore!

Labels Are for Cereal Boxes: Learning More about Your Sexual Orientation

During his time as lead singer of the band R.E.M., Michael Stipe was constantly asked about his sexual orientation, as people were quite fascinated with him and curious about what he might say. A setting of boundaries with others about his personal experience of his sexuality: "My feeling is that labels are for canned food. I am what I am—and I know what I am."

And truly, there are a tremendous number of labels you can use to describe your sexual orientation and gender identities. Some of these labels, like "gay" and "lesbian," have been around for a long time. Some of these labels have been reclaimed as terms of empowerment, like "queer" and even "fag." Some of these labels may be projected onto you by cisgender and straight people—or even people in the LGBTQ community—and can be frustrating, limiting, or even downright disrespectful. You may have also heard people complain about the changing language the LGBTQ community uses: "What?! Another term I need to know? I can't keep up with the alphabet soup!"

It is perfectly fine to have a lot of feelings about labels—or terms—and to explore them, claim them, challenge them, or implode them. In the introduction, I explained why I use "queer" and "trans" as umbrella terms—just as the term "LGBTQ" can encompass many gender and sexual orientation identities. It may seem weird that all of these terms are lumped together, because there are many differences between them. For instance, the term "sexual orientation" refers to the attractions you have to other people. Lots of people think that sexual orientation refers only to queer folks, and you may even feel uncomfortable sometimes when people talk about your sexual orientation. News alert: straight folks have a sexual orientation too! You may not feel that great talking about your sexual orientation, because you feel singled out to talk about this one part of your identity, when straight folks don't ever have to talk about their sexual orientation because it is just seen as "normal." Some folks prefer to use the term "affectional orientation," asserting that sexual attraction does not define who you are.

In addition, many folks are not aware that there are all sorts of sexual orientations that don't always seem to fit underneath the LGBTQ umbrella. Sure, words like "lesbian," "bisexual," "gay," and "queer" seem pretty straightforward. Lesbians tend to be attracted to people who identify as women, and gay people tend to be attracted to people who identify as men. Bisexual people tend to be attracted to many genders (some people do not like the term "bisexual" because it implies there are two genders; more on that in a moment). "Queer" truly is an umbrella term for all of these identities, but the key is that "queer" is a term that was previously used as an epithet and has been reclaimed to denote a politicized identity. Queer can denote attractions to one or many genders. Similarly, there are terms that refer to many attractions: "omnisexual" and "pansexual" people tend to be attracted to all genders, whereas "polysexual" people feel attracted to many genders. Contrasting to bisexuality, "monosexual" people tend to be attracted to one gender, and can be straight or queer.

But what about the term "questioning"? Many people might think this term means only that someone is confused about their sexual orientation or that it applies only to people who are just beginning to explore their sexual orientation. But if you think about it, sexual orientation can be quite fluid over the life span. Who and what you are drawn to in life can deepen, change, morph, and shift at any moment. A questioning identity is truly important, as it can also denote and recognize the very human part of you that explores your sexual orientation over your entire life span.

In other words, you can identify as queer *and* questioning. As you consider looking for ways you might not exactly fit into a sexual orientation box, let's consider sexual attraction and sexual behavior. Many people confuse these or think they mean the same thing. To clarify, your sexual attractions are how you *feel*, whereas sexual behavior is what you *do*. For some, at different times, sexual attraction and sexual behavior align—say, a gay man feels attracted to people who identify as men, and those are his sexual partners. For others or at other times, attraction and behavior don't align at all. A lesbian may be attracted to people who are women but occasionally enjoy sex with people who identify as men. Finally, we should acknowledge people who identify as *asexual*—they tend to not want to engage in sexual behavior, and they may or may not feel strong attractions to others.

Confused? Don't be! Sexual attraction and behavior can be normal and awesome parts of who you are, and your resilience in these areas is linked to how much you let yourself explore them. Again, all of these identities are not only healthy and normal, but also integral to your resilience as you learn more and more about who you are. To explore your sexual orientation further, check out the following resilience practice.

RESILIENCE PRACTICE: Exploring Your Sexual Orientation

The goal of this practice is to reflect on your sexual orientation and the term or terms you may use to describe yourself, then check off the sexual orientation identities that you feel most apply to you. These include some common terms, like "lesbian" (women who love women), "gay" (men who love men), "bisexual" (people who love more than one gender), "queer" (people who may fit into one of the previous categories, but who are reclaiming a previous epithet as a positive term; also used as an umbrella term), and "questioning" (people who are exploring their sexual orientation). There are some terms that may seem newer to you as well, such as "asexual" (people who do not experience sexual attraction and/or who have romantic relationships only), "monosexual" (people who experience attractions to one gender only; this can refer to straight or queer people), "omnisexual" or "pansexual" ("omni" and "pan" mean "all," so these are people who can experience love with all genders), "polysexual" ("poly" means "many," so these are people who experience love with many genders), and "same gender loving" (a phrase emerging from African American communities, indicating racial/ethnic and sexual orientation pride). (Note: This is just a partial list of the most commonly used terms.) It's OK to check more than one identity. And if you feel that none of the terms resonates with you, you get to be creative and make up your own terms (like "queerly straight") and define them, filling in the blanks.

☐ Asexual	☐ Pansexual
☐ Bisexual	☐ Polysexual
☐ Gay	☐ Queer
☐ Lesbian	☐ Questioning
☐ Monosexual	☐ Same-gender loving
☐ Omnisexual	

☐ _____

☐ _____

☐ _____

☐ _____

☐ _____

What was it like for you to complete this exercise? Was there one term that clearly feels good to use to sum up your sexual orientation? Or did you check several terms? You may have learned some new terms that feel good to use to describe your sexual orientation, or the terms offered may have been sorely insufficient and using your own self-generated descriptors feels more true to you. Regardless, naming things is important, and when it comes to sexual orientation pride, using the terms that feel best to you increases your resilience.

Never be bullied into silence. Never allow yourself to be made a victim.
Accept no one's definition of your life, but define yourself.

—Harvey Fierstein, White, Jewish, gay actor

"I Am My Own Gender": Taking a Closer Look at Your Gender Journey

Next, let's talk about gender. Society gets really hung up on gender. Right from the moment you are born, people applaud: "Yay, it's a boy!" or "Yay, it's a girl!" No one says, "Yay, it's a baby!" And so the gender training begins right from birth. You are taught the things you are supposed to do because you were assigned a certain sex (usually male or female, even though there are way more than just two!) at birth, and you are supposed to behave according to your assigned gender identity as boy or girl and man or woman. Within this sex and gender binary, there is little wiggle room. It's a shame, because many people believe there are as many gender identities as there are all the humans who have ever existed on the earth—essentially, that your own gender identity and how you express that gender is unique to yourself in the world.

However, when you step outside of those assigned-sex and gender boxes, then you get criticized, slammed, or simply encouraged to get back into line with your sex and gender assignment. These experiences can negatively influence how you see yourself and come to know your gender identity. The resilience you have developed to deal with these challenges, in addition to the resilience you can continue to cultivate in managing these experiences, really matters. It is as important for you to identify your gender identity as it is to choose the language *you* want to use to describe your sexual orientation identity. This journey of exploration can lead you through many emotions as well. In many ways, the emotions that come up as you begin to explore your gender identity make sense, as gender training can be very intense at all stages of life, and especially at earlier ages.

When I talk about exploring gender identity, let's be clear: I am not talking about only trans people doing this. Sure, things can get quite intense when you are trans, especially when you are exploring your gender while having to navigate anti-trans messages. And it is important for *everyone* to look deeply into their gender to see what identities, internalized beliefs, and social messages are there, as these can enhance or take away from your resilience. Again, your resilience increases the most when you have the space and supports you need to explore what your gender is, and when you are able to define your gender for yourself.

Part of your gender journey can include not only being able to define your own gender identities for yourself, but also having others value and respect those identities. Cisgender people are those who tend to agree with the sex they were assigned at birth and the gender identity that society says goes along with that sex. For instance, a cisgender man is someone whose assigned sex is male and whose gender identity is male, whereas a trans person may have an assigned sex that she does not agree with, such as a trans woman who was assigned male at birth by society but who identifies as a woman. Some trans people engage in a social transition, in which they want different names or pronouns to be used when referring to them; other trans people also want a medical transition, in which they access different medical interventions like hormones and surgery.

Under the trans umbrella there are also many gender identities, and many of these can range over the life span. For instance, some folks have adopted the term "genderqueer" to express that their gender is neutral, changing, or many genders at once or at different times. Genderqueer people may want some medical interventions, or none at all. Some people feel really strongly about identifying as a transsexual person, as they have typically engaged in some medical interventions—but not necessarily. Culture shapes the use of language as well. For instance, people of color began using terms such as "masculine of center" to designate their gender identity, falling somewhere on the trans spectrum. On the other hand, there are many trans people who want people to call them a man or woman and really do not feel strongly about a "trans" identity.

Although gender identity is different from sexual orientation, there is some overlap. Gender is also pretty fluid throughout one's life. Sure, you may see yourself with a fairly constant gender identity, but you may notice little changes and tweaks over time in terms of your gender expression, gender roles, gender attitudes, and gender beliefs. You may internally feel more "feminine" in terms of your gender identity, but you may feel drawn to express your gender in a more "masculine" manner. I put these words in quotes, as they are very binary and can be insufficient to truly describe the actual range of gender identities and gender expressions. On the other hand, some parts of your gender may be more affirmed by society—say, if you were assigned a male sex at birth and express your gender in a "masculine" way by wearing suits and ties at work, but you actually feel more like *yourself* when you go to work in clothes considered more "feminine." Over the course of my life, I have moved from a more androgynous gender expression (meaning staying away from the gender binary of gender expression) to a more feminine gender expression (like wearing dresses) as my gender identity has become more nonbinary and genderqueer. So really, "genderqueer femme" sums up my gender identity and gender expression perfectly *for me*.

You can see that gender identity and gender expression can be fluid. Just as with your sexual orientation, you may have many terms that are meaningful to you, or just one term, or no terms. Among the gender identities I'll be mentioning, there may be some terms you recognize that refer to people who were assigned a sex at birth that aligns with the gender they are (cisgender). The rest of the terms refer to people who were assigned a sex at birth with which they do not agree, in terms of their gender (trans and transgender are common "umbrella" terms for this community). Some trans people experience a binary gender—like "man," "woman," or "MTF" (male-to-female), "FTM" (female-to-male), and "transsexual." These last three terms can also indicate trans people who want to access medical services as part of their gender identity and expression, such as hormones and surgery.

There are other terms that specifically denote a rejection of the gender binary and embrace gender fluidity, such as "genderqueer," "nonbinary," "genderfluid," "genderblender," "gender neutral," "gender nonconforming," and "gender variant." "Bigender" also refers to people who experience a collection of multiple genders within their gender identity, "pangender" refers to people who experience all genders within themselves, and "polygender" refers to experiencing many genders. "Two-spirit" refers to trans people who have indigenous, Native American, and/or First Nations racial/ethnic backgrounds. Some terms specifically denote gender expression, such as "boi," which can be used by cisgender or trans people to describe a more masculine gender expression. "Crossdresser" refers to a person who expresses gender in a way that does not traditionally fit in with social conceptions of the gender binary. "Transmasculine" and "transfeminine" have emerged as terms to move away from some of the gender binary under the trans umbrella to denote gender expression. You can use the next resilience practice to further reflect on your own gender related to these terms.

RESILIENCE PRACTICE: Exploring Your Gender

The goal of this resilience practice is to explore your own gender identity and gender expression and identify the words that make you feel good. Check off the words that fit who you see yourself as being. If none seems to fit, create and write your own in the blanks!

- ☐ Bigender
- ☐ Boi
- ☐ Cisgender
- ☐ Crossdresser
- ☐ Female-to-male (FTM)
- ☐ Gender neutral
- ☐ Gender nonconforming
- ☐ Gender variant
- ☐ Genderblender
- ☐ Genderfluid

- ☐ Genderqueer
- ☐ Male-to-female (MTF)
- ☐ Pangender
- ☐ Polygender
- ☐ Trans
- ☐ Transfeminine
- ☐ Transgender
- ☐ Transmasculine
- ☐ Transsexual
- ☐ Two-spirit

- ☐ _____
- ☐ _____
- ☐ _____
- ☐ _____

Being able to name your own sexual orientation with words that fit your own identity contributes to resilience, and the same applies to your gender identity and gender expression. No one gets to tell you how you identify your gender—that is up to you. And the way you may identify your gender can be fluid and changeable. As you read through the list and checked off words, you may have seen one clear word or phrase that fit you. Or you may have selected several. Or maybe none of the words fit, and you created your own words. Notice which words make you feel empowered—that is what affirming your gender identity and increasing your resilience is all about.

[There is] wonderful news: news that gendered options can continue to explode, that the chefs in the kitchen of gender are creating new and imaginative specials every day. That we, all of us, are the chefs. Hi. Have a whisk.

—S. Bear Bergman, White, Jewish storyteller and gender jammer

Sharing about Your Gender and Sexual Orientation with Others

You may wear your gender and sexual orientation identities right on your sleeve—loudly and proudly communicating who you are to others. Some folks are open to hearing questions about their identities and enjoy talking about these parts of themselves. For others, these identities are way more private; they like to keep these parts of themselves to themselves. Still others might feel they are constantly intruded upon by other people because of how people perceive their sexual orientation and gender identities, and these intrusions—even if out of good intent and simple curiosity—feel like disrespectful, chronic, and draining experiences that can sap your resilience.

In addition, depending on other cultural identities you may have (I will talk more about these identities in Chapter 2), you may feel differently about communicating with others depending on the place or setting in which you are asked. For instance, you may feel open to talking about your identity in LGBTQ spaces, but less comfortable talking about these parts of you at work or in school. In addition to your feelings changing based on where you are and the people around you, how you communicate to others about your queer and trans identities can change over time. For example, I feel pretty open about my queer identity as a person of color with my family now, but when I first came out as a South Asian, multiracial person, I did not want to talk about these parts of my identities with my family. I was in the beginning of exploring these parts of myself, and it did not feel good to be pressed by them to define myself.

Essentially, fluidity applies not just to how you explore and experience your queer and trans identities. Deciding how you want—or don't want—to express your identities can be fluid and shifting as well. The thing is, having what's called an "elevator speech" about who you really are can be really helpful for when you *want* to communicate to others. Elevator speeches are short blurbs explaining ideas or concepts—basically, what you could communicate to someone else in an elevator in the time it takes to travel from the ground floor to the top floor of a building. My elevator speech about my identities goes like this (you will notice I have multiple identities):

I love being queer, South Asian, multiracial, and nonbinary. Being queer means I have attractions to many genders. "Queer" is an empowering term for me, because it connects me to a vibrant community of fellow queer and trans folks who are working for justice and liberation of all people.

You will notice that your elevator speech can change over time, but it is a good thing to check in with, as it can help you set boundaries and expectations of how you want to be treated. Explore your own elevator speech in the next resilience practice.

RESILIENCE PRACTICE: Bring Your Elevator Speech to Life!

Try writing your own elevator speech here, and notice which parts feel easy to write about and which feel more difficult. You might want to write about your sexual orientation *and* gender identities, and/or add some other important parts of who you are (like a young person, person with a disability, or working-class background):

_____

_____

_____

_____

_____

_____

Did the words come to you easily? How did it feel to write your elevator speech? Was it easy, rolling right off your tongue? Or did it feel more challenging to get started and communicate?

The key with your elevator speech is to stay connected with who you know yourself to be, and to value who you are so you can communicate that to other people.

Essentially, you want to let folks know how you expect to be treated when you get asked questions, especially when dealing with cisgender and straight folks who may not have ever thought about *their own* sexual orientation and gender identities. Here are some examples of what you might say when you feel empowered and good about sharing your identities with someone else:

- I would love to share about what my [insert your awesome identities here] means to me. [Insert your elevator speech.]

- I am just beginning to explore my [insert your awesome identities], and appreciate your support in asking me about these.

- Sure—happy to share about my [insert your awesome identities]. I would love to hear what your identities mean to you as well.

Of course, there are the times it feels a little weird to get asked certain questions. You will recognize these instances, as your gut will start sounding a mini-alarm and call for you to consider your boundaries of what is comfortable and not comfortable to share. Therefore, it is good to be prepared to communicate to others the boundaries you have about what is OK for them to ask you, as well as what is not OK. In these situations, take time to check in with your feelings and then communicate them to others; for example:

- I hear you asking about my [insert your awesome identities], but please know it's OK to ask _____ and it's not OK to ask _____.

- When I hear you asking about my [insert your awesome identities], although I trust your good intentions, I feel uncomfortable talking about this with you because _____.

- I don't feel comfortable answering that/those questions. Let's talk about something else.

Notice that the last example is perfectly fine to share. "No" is a word, a full sentence, and a perfectly awesome response with boundaries. Remember, *you* get to decide what feels good to share and not share. The next resilience practice (which you can download in worksheet form from http://www.newharbinger.com/39461) helps you think about how you can set boundaries with others who might not respect your identities.

RESILIENCE PRACTICE: Setting Boundaries about Your Identities

The goal of this resilience practice is to explore how you can set boundaries about your own identities with others. Sometimes you experience situations in which you cannot assume someone's good intentions when they ask questions about your identities. For instance, you might feel bullied or harassed, which can really decrease your resilience. You may have experienced so much oppression—or you may have been so conditioned to not stand up for yourself as a queer or trans person—that it is difficult to notice when you feel uncomfortable with something someone has said to you about your identities. Your gut is like your personal alarm system, signaling you when something may be wrong and you need to pay attention. Here are a few statements you can make in these situations—possible boundary-setting conversations for when your alarm system goes off.

- It is not OK for you to ask me that question. Please do not do that again.

- You used a wrong name and incorrect pronouns to refer to me. I expect you to use my correct name and pronouns.

- You assumed I had a man as a partner, and that is not OK to do.

- Being [insert your awesome identities] is important to me, and I expect you to treat me with respect in that regard.

Take time to think of an instance when you've experienced overt negativity and discrimination related to your gender and sexual orientation identities, when you needed to establish boundaries. Recall where this happened, or the person this has happened with, and remember how you felt. Now think of possible responses to protect yourself and your resilience. Write down a few boundary-setting conversations you could have with that person or in that situation:

_____

_____

_____

_____

_____

_____

How did it feel to write about boundary setting? Was it easy, challenging, or somewhere in between? No matter how it was for you, it is so important to practice these boundary-setting conversations in advance so they come naturally when the situation arises. With more practice and attention to your identities boundaries, your gut will then sound a louder alarm to take action because you are *paying attention* and tuned in to yourself. As I've said, some LGBTQ people and people of various diverse backgrounds and identities experience such consistent and repeated discrimination that they get used to hearing people say such things to them; they become numb to it, or even just laugh it off—"They don't really mean what they said."

It definitely is not fun to have to prepare elevator speeches for these situations. However, the more you practice them, the better you get at it. You feel more empowered—and your resilience increases. Often, you are just living your life when these microaggressions and macroaggressions happen. They can hit you out of the blue and take you from having a fabulous day to feeling despair and hopelessness. In these difficult situations, it is key to not just bounce back from a difficult experience, pushing it behind you. You want to be prepared for the next one. The next resilience practice helps you explore the specific tough situations in which you have needed to be resilient as a queer or trans person.

///

RESILIENCE PRACTICE: Understanding Adversity and Resilience as an LGBTQ Person

The goal of this resilience practice is to reflect on some of the hard things in life—adversity—that you have had to go through as a queer or trans person and to understand what resilience looks like in your own life. Think back: What is the most recent really hard thing you've gone through as an LGBTQ person? Did family members or friends reject you? Did you feel confused about your gender or sexual orientation? What else did you experience (or are you currently experiencing) as an LGBTQ person that is hard? Write briefly about those experiences:

_____

_____

_____

_____

What you just wrote describes the adversity you have had to bounce back from, showing your resilience as an LGBTQ person. Now think about what helped you get through that hard time and get back to feeling like your usual self again. Was it something you believed about yourself or a person? Describe what helped you here:

_____

_____

_____

_____

///

It may have been painful to write about adversity and tough times as a queer or trans person. Or you may have felt some distance from the experience because it was a long time ago. For now, just notice what you felt in writing about the hard times. Next, reflect on what it was like to write about your resilience in the face of that adversity. Did you feel proud of yourself? Did you feel impressed? Is the situation a current one that is ongoing and still difficult to be resilient to as an LGBTQ person? Again, notice how you feel about starting to understand your own resilience as an LGBTQ person and what actions might express that resilience. When these everyday challenges confront you, especially when no one is around to stand up for you, remember that as a queer and trans person you are worthy of respect, value, support, and love.

Remembering Your Value: Unearthing Internalized Heterosexism and Transnegativity

A big challenge to your resilience can really come down to the thoughts, messages, and beliefs in your head that you have internalized from the outside world. This process of internalizing not-so-great ideas about your sexual orientation and gender identities is variously referred to as "internalized oppression," "internalized heterosexism," and "internalized transnegativity." Sometimes you will hear the terms "internalized homophobia," "internalized transphobia," "internalized biphobia," and so on. But if you think about it, when people think, do, or say bad things about your gender and sexual orientation identities, it is discrimination—not fear—and it is important to identify it as discrimination. Sure, someone may be super oppressive toward us and experience some fear of us, but their oppression is more accurately identified as discrimination. I am using these terms—"heterosexism" and "transnegativity"—intentionally to call out what is *actually* going on in these instances.

Building resilience to internalized oppression entails identifying those messages—and sometimes these can be buried so deep inside of us that we do not even realize we have these negative beliefs. Again, your internalized negative beliefs can shift and change over different contexts and over your life span. Clearly, the more space these negative thoughts take up in your mind, the less room you have to explore who you are and to value your unique identities.

To get a visual of this process, picture your mind as a cup. The more internalized oppression there is in this cup, the less room you have for the positive beliefs, knowledge, and resilience you need to deal with the adversity that might come your way. You want to fill up your cup with lots of good and true thoughts about being LGBTQ to crowd out the more negative messages when they are imposed on you, because then there is simply no room for those messages to take up space in your mind.

Before you begin probing your mind to identify those internalized beliefs, let's think about all of the things you love and cherish about your sexual orientation and gender identities. Starting with the positives can be a first step to identify more and more things that are good about queer and trans people. I asked Jamie Roberts, a White queer trans woman, what she loved the most about herself; here's what she said about her identities:

> I love being queer and trans because I get to see the world and the people in it in a way I could never have if I were not. Because I had to love my whole self in order to survive and it challenged me to be a better, stronger human being with more empathy and will. Because I have freedom from the constricting confines of conventional gender expression and sexuality. Because I made friends and found family who see me in my entirety and would not abandon me to any difficulty. Because I understand now what is real love.

—Jamie Roberts, White, trans woman, filmmaker and attorney

Jamie's self-description can not only take up space in her mind, filling up her cup, but also be a source of strength for her to come back to when she hears or experiences ideas to the contrary. Complete the next resilience practice to explore how you appreciate your own gender and sexual orientation identities.

RESILIENCE PRACTICE: Affirming Your Gender and Sexual Orientation

The goal of this exercise is to affirm your own gender and sexual orientation. Take a moment to think about your own gender and sexual orientation identities. What would you say you appreciate about yours? You may have a lot to say—that's great! Keep writing! If you are struggling to get clear on what you like about your identities, that is OK too. Try writing a few words or bullet points, rather than full sentences. No pressure. Sometimes it can help to step outside of yourself. Then you can see things that are amazing about you that you do not even acknowledge. Think about what the people you trust would say. And if there are no people in your life right now whom you trust with your sexual orientation and gender identities, imagine you are your own supportive and awesome parent. From that perspective, what might you say?

_____

_____

_____

_____

_____

Now take a deep breath. How cool is it to spend a little time highlighting what is good and unique about you? Take in those positive messages—and then work on *believing* those messages. (That is really what this entire book is about: the journey to accepting and loving who you are.) And—news flash!—these are the types of messages that queer and trans people *should* be hearing and internalizing from the world. Until that world full of trans- and queer-affirming messages is ever-present, it is your job to make sure you create that supportive world inside of your mind. It's kind of like your mind has been "colonized" with these negative beliefs, and your resilience is very connected to showing them the door and externalizing these beliefs.

Being gay is natural. Hating gay is a lifestyle choice.

—John Fugelsang, White, straight, cigender
Christian activist

Challenging Myths and Stereotypes about Being Queer and Trans

Now that you have a good start on remembering your goodness, let's do another dig, to identify those negative beliefs. In these practices, you are shining a light into the hidden corners of your mind—challenging yourself to look beyond what you assume you know and feel about being queer and trans. To do this, it is helpful to consider all of the myths and stereotypes about being queer and trans that get promoted in the media and bandied about in communities and even within your family. Explore some of these anti-LGBTQ messages in the following resilience practice.

RESILIENCE PRACTICE: What Have You Heard about Being LGBTQ?

The goal of this resilience practice is to identify what you have heard in the way of messages, myths, and just stuff that does not help you feel good about your gender and sexual orientation—and then to challenge those messages. In the following list, you may recognize some messages you've heard from people you know, or that you've been exposed to over time. Check off the ones that you apply to your life. These messages can vary based on the geographical region you were raised in and the religion or spiritual practices you were raised with, among many other circumstances. Sometimes you can experience a mixture of messages that may *seem* positive but actually are negative—or vice versa. Feel free to use the blanks at the end of the list to fill in messages you may have heard about queer and trans people that you know are just not right:

- ☐ LGBTQ people are choosing to be LGBTQ, and they can choose not to be.
- ☐ There are only two genders.
- ☐ Being straight or cisgender is normal, and LGBTQ people are abnormal.
- ☐ People are LGBTQ because they were taught to be.
- ☐ LGBTQ are that way because they were sexually abused.
- ☐ Queer and trans people should not be parents because they will harm their children.
- ☐ Being LGBTQ is a sin and against God.
- ☐ LGBTQ people cannot develop healthy relationships.
- ☐ LGBTQ people will always be unhappy.
- ☐ LGBTQ people are promiscuous.
- ☐ LGBTQ people are confused and can be cured—they just have not met the right person yet.
- ☐ LGBTQ people can't know who they are unless they have had sex with the right person.
- ☐ LGBTQ issues should not be taught in schools, as children will learn to be LGBTQ.
- ☐ Being LGBTQ means choosing a hard life.
- ☐ If you are around an LGBTQ person, they will be interested in having sex with you.
- ☐ Being LGBTQ is just a phase.
- ☐ _____
- ☐ _____
- ☐ _____
- ☐ _____

Whew! These myths and stereotypes are hard to read, one right after the other, or to write down from your own experience or internalized beliefs. It's normal to feel some anger, frustration, or fear come up as you read through these. Maybe you checked several you have heard, just a few, or none at all. The point of this exercise is to start examining the messages you have heard and identifying how much space those myths and stereotypes take up in your mind. If you did check a few—or many—of these myths and stereotypes, take some time to write here how those social messages affected you in terms of how you think and feel about your gender and sexual orientation identities:

_____

_____

_____

_____

_____

_____

Just like the elevator speech you explored earlier in the chapter—for which you thought about what you might say in a situation where you feel disrespected, challenged, or judged about your identities—it is important to name the social messages you receive about your sexual orientation and gender identities and then to challenge how you might have internalized those messages. When you hear something about LGBTQ people in general—or about your own identities—you can ask yourself the following questions:

- Is this something that is *actually* true?

- Is this something *I want to believe* about myself and/or my community?

- Does this message make me feel better about myself?

These three questions can quickly help you distinguish the messages that are good to take in and nourishing to your resilience from those intended to make you doubt yourself, feel bad, or believe things about yourself that are just not true.

Just to give you an idea of the influences these types of messages can have, and how you can internalize them, read through the list in the next resilience practice (which is also available as a worksheet at http://www.newharbinger.com/39461).

RESILIENCE PRACTICE: Internalizing LGBTQ-Affirming Messages

There are many wonderful messages you should have been hearing in relation to being queer and trans. Pay attention to how you feel when you read this list, and place a checkmark next to the messages you have heard and/or believe to be true. At the end of the list, there is space for you to write any further messages from the world you would have loved to hear about LGBTQ communities that are specific to you (like your multiple identities, cultural background, or anything else that is awesome about you as a queer or trans person!).

- ☐ Being LGBTQ is wonderful.

- ☐ There are multiple gender and sexual orientation identities—not just a few labels to be assigned by society.

- ☐ LGBTQ people come to know who they are in many different ways.

- ☐ LGBTQ people deserve respect, love, and understanding from their families, friends, and communities.

- ☐ LGBTQ people can create wonderful families of choice.

- ☐ LGBTQ people can be great parents if they choose to raise children.

- ☐ LGBTQ people have existed around the world across time and continents.

- ☐ LGBTQ people can have wonderful and healthy relationships.

- ☐ Being free to be yourself as an LGBTQ person can make you very happy.

- ☐ LGBTQ people deserve to have fulfilling and respectful sexual relationships if that is important to them.

- ☐ Because LGBTQ people have to deal with challenges related to being LGBTQ, they often have strengths and resilience that help them in other areas of their lives.

- ☐ The important contributions of LGBTQ people and communities should be taught in schools.

- ☐ LGBTQ people can be deeply religious and/or spiritual with no conflict between their identities, if that is important to them.

- ☐ LGBTQ people can explore their sexual orientation and gender identities over their lifetimes.

☐ _____

☐ _____

☐ _____

☐ _____

As you completed this resilience practice, you may have felt encouraged because you checked many LGBTQ-affirming messages. Or you may have felt discouraged because you had few checkmarks. However many you checked, keep working on the positive messages you still want to internalize to grow your resilience. Let any feeling of discouragement motivate you to get more support to grow your resilience (you will read more about this in Chapter 8). Just reading this workbook and completing the resilience practices will help you identify new positive messages that support your resilience—and even remind you of the many awesome and unique gifts you bring to the world as a queer or trans person.

In trans women's eyes, I see a wisdom that can only come from having to fight for your right to be recognized as female, a raw strength that only comes from unabashedly asserting your right to be feminine in an inhospitable world.

—Julia Serano, White, trans, feminist woman
and author

Doesn't the list in the preceding resilience practice feel better to read than the first one? Social messages and stereotypes are like the air you breathe. You may not notice how polluted the air feels, but LGBTQ people definitely deserve to breathe fresh, healthy air! This means that you can increase your resilience by realizing that the social air you breathe is unclean, but you can put on a resilience mask through which clean oxygen starts flowing because you take control of the messages you have internalized and counter these messages with the real truth about LGBTQ people—that being an LGBTQ person is a beautiful and wonderful thing! Do the next resilience practice to rate the areas in which your resilience is strong—and the areas you need to work on some more.

RESILIENCE PRACTICE: Shaping the Messages in Your Mind about Being LGBTQ

In this resilience practice, you explore internalized messages about being LGBTQ and how affirming those messages are. Read the following statements that explore how LGBTQ-affirming the messages are that you receive from yourself, others, and the world. For each, write an X or checkmark in the column indicating whether you agree, somewhat agree, or disagree with the statement.

Beliefs about Yourself:	Agree	Somewhat Agree	Disagree
Being LGBTQ is a good thing.			
I am lucky to be LGBTQ.			
I know a lot about myself as an LGBTQ person.			
Messages from Others:			
I deserve to have people in my life who support me as an LGBTQ person.			
I have people in my life who support me as an LGBTQ person.			
I have a community of LGBTQ people I reach out to in challenging times.			
Messages from the World:			
I am exposed to messages in the world that LGBTQ people are a valued and important part of society.			
I am aware of the organizations that are advocating for the rights of LGBTQ people.			
I am connected with media outlets (local, national, international) that are affirming of LGBTQ people.			
Totals:			

Add up the responses in each column. Do you mainly agree, somewhat agree, or disagree with the messages you have internalized related to yourself, others, and the world?

Now think about what you might need to do to internalize more positive messages about yourself as an LGBTQ person, such as reading LGBTQ-affirming literature such as books and blogs, connecting with LGBTQ community, getting support from cisgender and straight people who are LGBTQ-affirming, or meeting with a counselor. In the following space, write about what you need in order to internalize more LGBTQ-affirming messages (which naturally will increase your resilience).

_____

_____

_____

_____

Let's be gentle with ourselves and each other and fierce as we fight oppression.

—Dean Spade, trans activist, founder of
Sylvia Rivera Law Review Project

Resilience Wrap-Up

Queer and trans people can and should define their own gender and sexual orientation identities. These processes not only are a large part of your resilience but also help fill your mind with positive messages about who you are, so the negative messages cannot take up as much space. You can strengthen your resilience as an LGBTQ person through:

- Exploring your gender and sexual orientation identities

- Valuing your gender and sexual orientation identities

- Defining your gender and sexual orientation identities *for yourself*

- Identifying internalized negative messages about being LGBTQ and where they come from—places like family, school, and general society

- Challenging internalized negative messages through valuing your unique identities as an LGBTQ person

- Connecting with people who are affirming of LGBTQ people and support you in expressing your true self

Now that you have reflected further on your gender and sexual orientation identities, in Chapter 2 you will learn how these identities intersect with so many other parts of yourself—like race/ethnicity, class, disability—and with your experiences of resilience related to the intersections of these multiple identities.

You Are More Than Your Gender and Sexual Orientation

The wild thing about exploring your gender and sexual orientation and defining these identities for yourself is that as you continue to explore these two identities, you realize you are so much more than just these two! There are innumerable combinations, as I shared about my own identities in the introduction. You may identify as a:

- Latinx woman

- Gay man with a physical disability

- Bisexual man with a mental health disability

- Transmasculine person from a working-class background

- Bisexual, bigender, immigrant person raised in poverty, but now middle class

- Lesbian, Muslim, cisgender woman from an upper-class background, who is a U.S. citizen

You can see in just this short list that there are many possible combinations, and these are just a *few* of the huge number of various social identities. In this chapter, you'll build on the resilience that you identified related to being queer and/or trans, as you begin to explore what other social identities shape your resilience.

I remember how being young and black and gay and lonely felt. A lot of it was fine, feeling I had the truth and the light and the key, but a lot of it was purely hell.

—Audre Lorde, Black lesbian poet, writer, and activist

Intersections of Identity: Appreciating All of Who You Are

When you come out as an LGBTQ person, your resilience is challenged, as this typically entails struggling in a heteronormative and gender-binary world to embrace who you are. Similar processes happen with other parts of your identity, like your race or ethnicity, class background, disability, and religion or spirituality, among others. Ideally, all of your social identities would help you be more resilient throughout your life, so you feel good about yourself and have more freedom to pursue your hopes and dreams. But because there are conflicting messages about these social identities, you may be vulnerable to receiving messages that are not supportive of these important parts of who you are.

Socialization is the process people experience growing up of the cultural norms, rules, and guidelines of society. Just as you receive certain messages about being LGBTQ, you absorb a variety of messages about your other social identities. Sometimes these social identities are projected onto you from a very early age. For example, I am a multiracial person who grew up with a White mother and a father from northern India. I have said that I am a "racial Rorschach," because people project onto me what they think I am (and sometimes need me to be) in that moment. The tough thing about this is that I grew up in a distinctly Indian home, with smells of curry, Indian clothing, and the Sikh religion. At home I had a good deal of room and encouragement from my parents to explore my Indian and Sikh identities. However, when I left the house, the messages I received were that I was "half-Indian" and "half-White." My father wore a turban as a part of his religion, so I often was bullied about our family's being "terrorists." There were times I felt resilient to this bullying, but other times I did not feel much resilience at all.

My family was very educated, but also very poor. So, there was no money for new clothes, sports activities, new cars, travel, or other symbols of middle-class life. I received a good deal of bullying and messages from the world that I "wasn't right" in the eyes of the world. In addition, growing up in the Deep South of the United States, I received many messages about how I should act as a person who was assigned female at birth and raised as a girl. These messages included: be quiet, don't speak up too much, and look "pretty." These messages came from both the Western society where I grew up (New Orleans) *and* the Indian immigrant community, which meant I was receiving a *lot* of messages about being a girl.

You have your identity when you find out, not what you can keep your mind on, but what you can't keep your mind off.

—A. R. Ammons, White, cisgender man, poet

I share these messages from my childhood to help you start thinking about the messages you have learned related to your social identities. These messages can be positive, negative, or a combination. A good way to start developing your resilience in this regard is to think about how much you know about your identities besides your LGBTQ identity. The next resilience practice will get you started.

RESILIENCE PRACTICE: How Much Do I Know about My Own Identities?

The aim of this resilience practice is to start to name some of your various social identities. Sexual orientation and gender identity are included on this list so you can get a sense of how much you know about these two identities in relation to some of your other social identities. Write to the left side of the statement whether you "agree" (A), "somewhat agree" (SA), or "disagree" (D) that you know about this identity for you:

_____ Ability (emotional, physical, developmental)

_____ Age

_____ Geographic region

_____ Gender

_____ National origin

_____ Race or ethnicity

_____ Religion or spirituality, agnosticism, atheism

_____ Sexual orientation

_____ Social class

What did you notice as you went through this list of your social identities? Did you agree that you had more knowledge about some of your identities and not others? Are sexual orientation and gender identity something you know more or less about related to your other identities? Keep in mind the identities you know the least about, because you will be exploring more about each of these identities (except for gender and sexual orientation, which you explored in Chapter 1). Even for the social identities that you agreed you know a good deal about, there may be still more to learn in relation to increasing your resilience.

Before we continue exploring these social identities, let's talk about two words that can really influence your resilience: privilege and oppression. "Privilege" refers to your unearned advantages related to an identity. For instance, society grants cisgender privilege and straight privilege to people who are cisgender or straight. Cisgender people don't have to think about whether or not it is safe to use a bathroom, and straight people don't have to worry about being "out" or not to friends and family. When you have privilege you can be quite oblivious to it, as you have not done anything to earn it.

"Oppression" is the absence of these unearned advantages and the discrimination and denial of prejudice that people who have an oppressed identity experience. In each of the social identity categories listed earlier, there is a group that has privilege and a group that does not have privilege. The next resilience practice will help you explore some of your social identities related to privilege and oppression.

RESILIENCE PRACTICE: Identifying Your Unique Social Identity Privilege and Oppression Matrix

The goal of this resilience practice is to help you start seeing the intersections of your social identities with your experience of privilege and oppression. Circle or highlight the social identities in the table that apply to you, so you can visualize your individual mix of privilege and oppression social identities.

Social Identity	Privilege Status	Oppression Status
Ability Status	Able-bodied	Developmental/physical/ mental disability
Age	Adults	Children, adolescents, older adults
Education Level	Access to higher ed	High school/GED/ noncompletion
Geographic Region	Urban, suburban	Rural
Gender	Men, cisgender	Women, trans
National Origin	Western Europe, U.S. citizen	Asian, African, Eastern European, Latina/o, Middle Eastern

Race/Ethnicity	White	People of Color
Religion/Spirituality	Judeo-Christian	All others: Muslim, Eastern, Jewish, Pagan, secular, and so on
Sexual Orientation	Straight	LGBTQ, polyamorous
Social Class	Middle to upper class	Poverty to working class

As you circled your various identities, you may have noticed you have more social identities of privilege than you realized. These privileges may protect or buffer you from oppression as a queer and/or trans person, so your resilience may not be as challenged in these areas. For instance, a White, queer, cisgender man can be protected from some of the oppressive experiences associated with disability and sexual orientation, based on his racial/ethnic and gender privilege. On the other hand, you may notice you have many social identities associated with oppression. These identities can make you more vulnerable to decreased resilience, especially if you have many social identities associated with oppression. For example, a Latinx, lesbian, trans woman may experience oppression related to her sexual orientation, gender identity, and race/ethnicity.

Consider Will Mellman's description of his multiple identities:

For those who don't know anything more than what they see, I am a White man—a husband, father, brother, and son. Being a White man means, regardless of intent, I have access to certain spaces, privileges, and resources that others do not. However, unlike many White men, I recognize the privileges bestowed upon me, because I am also trans and Jewish. As a trans man, I am uniquely situated to understand the role of gender in a social and cultural context, having lived for twenty years as female. Being Jewish, which I claim as a cultural and ethnic identity, has also provided me a unique perspective from which to understand rejection and persecution simply based on one's beliefs. Both of these identities are easily concealable, regardless of my desires to outwardly claim membership in these groups. As a result, when I walk down the street, go to the supermarket, shop in a store, or even go to the doctor, I am a White man. This fact is not lost on me and, on a daily basis, shapes who I am.

—Will Mellman, White, Jewish, trans man, father

The good news is that the more you learn about your social identities—whether related to privilege or to oppression—the more you can build your resilience. You can use your unearned privilege to help yourself and other people who were not granted those privileges. You can be mindful that multiple oppressions can also translate into multiple sources of resilience you can use to challenge and overcome adversity.

Remember that the list of examples in the preceding resilience practice is not comprehensive; other identities, such as your primary language spoken and your immigration status, also come into play and influence your experience of resilience. In addition, as you explore describing these social identities, the examples' placement under the privilege or oppression heading may or may not relate to the experience you had. Let's use geographic region, for instance. You could be Native American and be raised in an urban environment, where there would not necessarily be more access to a Native American community who could support you. As with all things human, these concepts and ideas of privilege and oppression, so simply categorized in a list, are actually very complex and intersectional for your life and your resilience. As you proceed, keep in mind that you are considering these categories individually for now; later you will weave them all back together by the end of the chapter. Keep in mind you are also going in alphabetical order, and not in terms of the importance these identities may have for you.

People with impairments are disabled by their environments; or, to put it differently, impairments aren't disabling; social and architectural barriers are.

—Alison Kafer, professor of queer studies,
author of *Feminist, Queer, Crip*

Ability (Emotional, Physical, Developmental)

Ability refers to the presence or absence of emotional, physical, and/or developmental disabilities in a person's life. Many people think of the word "disability" and just think of functional impairment disabilities, like cerebral palsy, deafness, or visual impairment.

When we think about ability, it is important to consider cognitive and mental health disabilities too, such as depression, anxiety, bipolar, and dyslexia. Many of these disabilities are unnoticed and disrespected because they are not easily "seen" by society. This is very oppressive to people with cognitive or mental health disabilities, because they may feel they need to prove that they have the disability. Or they may feel they must hide or conceal this part of their identity because of internalized social stigma common with cognitive or mental health challenges. Queer and trans people, even if they do not have a disability, are often thrown into the disability category without their permission. For instance, mental health disabilities—and the way they are defined—can be really problematic, because as of this writing "gender dysphoria" is listed as a mental health disability in the *Diagnostic and Statistical Manual of Mental Disorders*. I do not like this categorization at all. What is not included in designations of disabilities is also problematic. Think about it. There is no "cisgenderism disorder," "heterosexism disorder," "racism disorder," or "classism disorder," among others, that could warrant a diagnosis! In our society, people tend to diagnose individual people, and not cultures of oppression, and that can be a challenge to our resilience, for sure.

In addition to physical, cognitive, and mental health disabilities, there are also developmental disabilities, which might include challenges with learning, reading, and communicating information. Somewhat like people with mental health challenges, those with developmental disabilities may have to advocate for themselves—or have strong advocates in their life—to help them receive needed services. No matter where you may be on the disability spectrum, you can use your own self-generated words to describe yourself, and these should be respected. For example, some disability rights activists describe themselves as "disabled" because they want their disabled identity to be a valued part of how they are seen in society. Other people dislike the word because they believe it implies that something has been done to them (an ability has been taken from them), rather than their disability being an important part of their identity.

Regardless, *you* get to decide. Just remember, if you do not *presently* have a physical, cognitive, or mental health disability, you may want to be mindful that this is likely a temporary state. As you age, your body changes as well, and you can move into a disability status. You can think of ability status as fluid, as you may have a permanent or temporary disability. If you do not have a present disability, you can still think about your ability identity and consider how to be an ally to people living with disabilities. Complete the next resilience practice to explore your thinking about your own ability and disability.

RESILIENCE PRACTICE: Exploring What Disability and Ability Mean

In this resilience practice, reflect on how disability and ability relate to your own identity. Read the following questions, take some time to think about your answers, and then write them down.

- Do you have a mental, cognitive, or physical health disability now?

- Do you know people with mental, cognitive, or physical health disabilities within your family, friends group, school, work, or other settings?

- Have you heard messages that being queer or trans is a mental, cognitive, or physical health disability?

_____

_____

_____

_____

How did it feel to respond to these questions? If you do not currently have a mental, cognitive, or physical health disability, did you think about how that might change in the future with age or other circumstances? As you considered others you know who may have a mental, cognitive, or physical health disability, what emotions came up? People who live with disabilities of all sorts constantly are given social messages that they are not normal and experience people feeling sorry for them. Consider what messages this sends to people living with disabilities, and the resilience they must develop to withstand these messages and develop a sense of pride and strength. Think about how society has also denigrated queer and/or trans identities as disabilities. For many people, it is really important to align their identities, both queer _and_ disabled, because society responds to both with similar negative messages.

I don't mind being different. Different is special! I think what matters most is what a person is like inside. And inside, I am happy. I am having fun. I am proud!

—Jazz Jennings, multiracial trans youth activist

Age

Most of us don't think of our age as a social identity, because it is a constant, slowly evolving fact of life. And as with disability, you may underestimate the possibility of experiencing oppression related to your age. But people do experience oppression based on their age, particularly early and late in the life span.

"Adultism" is a term for the oppression that children (up to age eleven) and adolescents and young adults (ages twelve to twenty-five) often experience from adults who have power and control over their lives. Adultism shapes young people's self-image and their ability to freely express their gender and sexual orientation identities. Children who experience gender nonconformity may have adults in their lives who forbid them to play with certain toys or wear certain clothes; adolescents who are awakening to their queer identities may feel it's not safe to share their identities with their family because they are afraid of getting kicked out of their home during high school or losing needed support during college. Adolescence is a very difficult time for many queer and trans people, as many feel they do not have the community, resources, or information they need to affirm their identities, and they may experience bullying, depression, suicidal ideation, and substance abuse.

Older folks (fifty and older) can also experience oppression related to their age, commonly termed "ageism." This ageism can include being viewed by society as having less to contribute, being seen as less attractive, and feeling invisible in a world that places great value on being or staying young. Older people who have spent their lives being out as a queer or trans person can develop disabilities as they age and need to rely on families that may not have been supportive of their being LGBTQ. Older people may also need assisted living and hospice care, where their pronouns and names are not respected—or where they feel like they need to conceal their LGBTQ identities for fear of being discriminated against, harmed, or neglected. Some LGBTQ people come out later in life and may feel they have missed a lot of living openly in their queer or trans identity and want to make up for lost time.

Queer and trans adults (from twenty-six to forty-nine) can be mindful of the privilege they enjoy with regard to age and, from this privileged position, reach out and support younger and older LGBTQ people in becoming more resilient to adultism and ageism challenges. When you help others, you end up helping yourself, too, because you develop a more positive and hopeful approach to life.

In the next resilience practice, you can reflect on your current age as an LGBTQ person and create some of the messages you *should* have been receiving about your life related to ages you have gone through. Every age you move through has its mix of wonderful experiences and challenges an LGBTQ person.

RESILIENCE PRACTICE: What's Age Got to Do with It?

In this resilience practice, explore what it means to you to be LGBTQ and to be the age that you are.

What thoughts and feelings do you have about being the age you are as an LGBTQ person?

_____

_____

_____

_____

What age-related strengths do you have as an LGBTQ person?

_____

_____

_____

_____

What age-related challenges have you faced as an LGBTQ person?

_____

_____

_____

_____

As you were writing, did you make the connection between your resilience and the age you are now? Do you feel proud of your age? If not, what type of support do you need to feel good about your age, and how can you grow your resilience related to your age right now? Don't wait to grow your age-related resilience; claim your age and all the amazing parts of being whatever age you are.

Geographic Region

Why bring up geography when talking about queer and trans resilience? Well, your geographic location can really shape your access to LGBTQ-affirming resources and community. If you are raised in rural areas, you might have had a distant queer or trans relative who moved away to the "big city." Suburban areas can have a lot of financial resources for schools, but may not have as many LGBTQ supports, like Gay-Straight Alliances (GSAs) or school personnel who are LGBTQ Safe Zone–trained. Urban environments can offer amazing things like a student body that's diverse in terms of race/ethnicity, immigrants, and LGBTQ students, but they often lack adequate funding for education.

Essentially, where you were raised can really influence how much resilience you have in relation to multiple social identities. Plus, you can be raised in one place that is anti-LGBTQ, and move to another to find more LGBTQ-affirming communities. Or you can be raised in a place that is LGBTQ-affirming, but then your job is relocated to a geographic region that is LGBTQ-negative. Some people must move every year for family, work, or to relieve financial stress, like families experiencing job loss and moving in with grandparents who may or may not understand LGBTQ identities.

To me, the interesting thing about geographic region is that it is often linked to what you consider *home*—whether this place was affirming of queer and trans people or not. The place we consider home can have a lot of meaning for us. You may go "home" for the holidays, then head back into an LGBTQ-negative geographic region, but the people you love and cherish still live in that home place. Where you grew up can have tremendous influence on your resilience; there could be many adversities to test your resilience, or many supportive people to help strengthen it, or a mix of both. Do the following resilience practice to explore where you were raised and what that was like for you.

RESILIENCE PRACTICE: Where Were You Raised?

In this resilience practice, you'll reflect on where you were raised in terms of geographic region and how that influenced your resilience as an LGBTQ person.

What specific challenges did you face as an LGBTQ person where you grew up?

_____

_____

What specific things nurtured your resilience as an LGBTQ person where you grew up?

_____

_____

Did you move around, or did you stay in the same geographic region? How did that experience affect your resilience as an LGBTQ person?

_____

_____

When you realized you were LGBTQ, did you have a LGBTQ community nearby or did you want to move closer to it? How did that affect your resilience?

_____

_____

//

I want to go down in history

in a chapter marked miscellaneous

because the writers could find

no other way to categorize me

In this world where classification is key

I want to erase the straight lines

So I can be me

>—Staceyann Chin, Jamaican-born, U.S. citizen, queer, cisgender woman, poet and activist

National Origin

No matter where you live, you have a national origin. This is somewhat related to geographic region, as it refers to the place you were born; national origin also can have a lot to do with race/ethnicity, which we'll explore next. National origin is an important social identity to consider, as LGBTQ people may be born in countries that are extremely anti-LGBTQ, or they may move to countries that are LGBTQ-affirming, in an effort to increase their resilience by being closer to queer and trans communities.

When you speak the language of the country in which you are living and appear to be a native, you may enjoy *national origin privilege*—the unearned advantages granted when people assume you "belong" in the country in which you live. Conversely, *national origin oppression* entails being discriminated against for your social identity when you appear to be from another country. You may be harassed about speaking the language with a nonnative accent or because of the way you look; you may feel you are treated as if you don't belong. The social identity of national origin may be linked in complicated ways to issues of immigration and having refugee or asylee status. In the next resilience practice you can explore these identities.

RESILIENCE PRACTICE: Reflecting on Your National Origin

The goal of this resilience practice is to get you thinking about your national origin. Consider the following questions and respond:

- Are you treated like you belong in the country in which you live?

- Do people think or assume you are originally from another country?

- Think about your family (however you define this family—family of choice and/or family of origin) and their national origin. How has their privilege in this regard—or their oppression—affected your identity and resilience as an LGBTQ person?

_____

_____

_____

_____

Writing about your national origin may surprise you; the messages can really vary. Certain groups of immigrants to the United States are held in high regard; other immigrant groups are held in disregard and experience tremendous oppression. National origin can vary for different generations, too. For instance, my mom's family (White, Scottish, Irish) has been in the United States for many generations; my dad (Indian) was an immigrant to this country. My mom never experienced anyone thinking she shouldn't be here or didn't belong in this country, whereas my dad was perpetually treated as a foreigner even when he had been in the country for several decades. They had quite different experiences of privilege and oppression related to their national origin.

In other words, it is a privilege to ignore the consequences of race in [the world].

—Tim Wise, White, cisgender male activist

Race and Ethnicity

Your race or ethnicity is another complicated social identity. People make assumptions, and they'll project onto you the racial/ethnic identity they assume for you, mostly in an effort to determine what that may mean about who you are as a person. Many people cannot hide their race/ethnicity, whereas they may be able to conceal their gender identity and sexual orientation identities. Because many of us come to know our LGBTQ identity only over time (such as experiencing attraction, expressing gender), our racial/ethnic identity—generally known to us from early childhood—can be a powerful and dominant influence.

Queer and trans people commonly hear questions like "When did you first know you were [insert LGBTQ identity]?" But because race/ethnicity is generally a more visible identity, you rarely hear a question like "When did you first know you were [insert racial/ethnic identity]?"

Because race/ethnicity is so visible, societal responses related to privilege and oppression can be quite intense. For instance, people of color experience racism and learn to anticipate racial microaggressions and macroaggressions, and then potentially shift how they think, look, feel, and communicate so they "fit in" with the dominant group—usually White folks. As people of color must contend with intergenerational experiences of racism as well, they commonly internalize negative messages about their own race/ethnicity. For instance, Asian American/Pacific Islanders might refuse to see physicians who share their own identity, preferring a White physician. Families of color may teach their children internalized racism as well, encouraging their children to meet a White norm of society and missing the opportunity to instill racial/ethnic pride, which is a major factor in resilience for both cisgender and LGBTQ people of color.

On the other side of the coin, just as people of color experience undeserved disadvantages related to race/ethnicity, White people experience unearned advantages. Sure, White people may not be explicitly racist or have participated in racist acts, but covert and embedded racism can sneak into your language and communication, in addition to the places you work, go to school, and play. Thus over time a White, Western "norm" or "majority" way of thinking has been established in our institutions, whereby certain racial groups are valued if they hew to that White norm, and those who do not are judged as resistant, lazy, or not good enough in comparison.

White privilege has its costs, however—not only to society as a whole, but also to White people themselves. Because of the legacy and history of racism, White people may not develop relationships with people of color and be exposed to the dynamic beauty of world cultures in all its variety.

Many people feel intensely uncomfortable talking about privilege and oppression in general, so they avoid it. When it comes to race/ethnicity, the silence can be even more pronounced—and when the issues are unavoidable, the debate can become quite heated. But the thing is, your resilience as a queer or trans person is imperatively linked to knowing yourself—*all* of your identities—and that includes your race/ethnicity. Research has shown that queer and trans people of color can be more resilient when they have *not only LGBTQ pride, but also racial/ethnic pride* (Singh & McKleroy, 2011; Singh, 2013). For LGBTQ people of color, exploring and digging out of ways they have internalized negative beliefs about themselves related to racism is crucial to strengthening their resilience. White LGBTQ people can be allies and stand up against all forms of racism by realizing that although they may not have created the pervasive structural racism in society, they can certainly be part of the solution by listening to and valuing the perspectives and experiences of LGBTQ people of color. In the next resilience practice, you'll further explore your race/ethnicity as an LGBTQ person.

RESILIENCE PRACTICE: Reflecting on Your Racial/Ethnic Identity as an LGBTQ Person

The goal of this resilience practice is to get you thinking about your racial/ethnic identity and your associated privilege or oppression experiences. Consider the following questions, then respond:

- Is your race/ethnicity related more to privilege, oppression, or a mix?

- Do you feel a sense of pride in your race/ethnicity? Why or why not?

- What kinds of messages have you received from your predominant racial/ethnic group about being LGBTQ?

- Overall, what does it mean to you to be an LGBTQ person of [insert your own racial/ethnic heritage or cultural background]?

_____

_____

_____

_____

As you completed this resilience practice, was it easy to write about your race/ethnicity, or challenging? Did you easily feel a sense of racial/ethnic pride, or did experiences of privilege or oppression related to your race/ethnicity make this more complicated? Were the messages you've received from your racial/ethnic group about your LGBTQ identity more positive, negative, some of both, or neutral? How do your answers to these questions influence how you feel about your overall race/ethnicity, gender, and sexual orientation identities? These questions are important, because, again, you increase your resilience when you can experience a sense of pride in your identities and also understand the complicated intersections of privilege and oppression that come with them.

Catholic guilt. I was raised Catholic. And somehow that whole idea, or that internal chatter, all started to talk to me, and say, "This is what happens. This is God's way of punishing you. You transitioned. You're an abomination. This is God's way of telling you He doesn't approve." It was very hard to bear.

—Cecilia Chung, Chinese American, HIV/AIDS and trans advocate

Religion, Spirituality, Agnosticism, and Atheism

Religion and spirituality can be vital social identities for LGBTQ people, as religious and spiritual values can be sources of coping and resilience. For those for whom religion/spirituality are important, it can also feel like a double-edged sword because they can experience so much discrimination based on their gender and sexual orientation identities. Queer and trans people have been rejected from churches, temples, gurdwaras, mosques, and other places of worship just because they are LGBTQ. On the other hand, there are religious/spiritual institutions that openly welcome and support LGBTQ people and become communities they can rely on during important events in life, like marriage, raising children, and death. The supportive religious/spiritual communities can even take the place of families who have rejected LGBTQ people, so it can be very healing for LGBTQ people to also be religious/spiritual.

At the same time, it is also important to acknowledge and support atheist and agnostic identities. These social identities are no less legitimate or valuable than other religious/spiritual identities, and often those who identify as atheist and agnostic feel minimized and invisible in society that is typically quite Judeo-Christian in its institutions and values. Atheist and agnostic people may have a coming-out process similar to what they went through with their LGBTQ identity. They may feel they have to choose carefully whom they disclose their identity to and consider the consequences for their relationships with family, friends, school settings, and workplaces when they come out. It is a different type of "closet"; however, this social rejection can multiply the experiences of isolation for LGBTQ atheist and agnostic people.

As is also true of the general population, there are LGBTQ people who practice less-well-known and less-accepted religions and spiritual traditions. These people may feel their resilience is challenged in this area by social stigma and ignorance. For instance, LGBTQ Muslims experience Islamophobia, hearing stereotypes and judgments that their religion is "terrorist," when Islam is a very peaceful religion. People who identify as Pagan or Wiccan may also feel their religious/spiritual practices are stereotyped as "evil." Therefore, under the religious/spiritual umbrella of social identity there is also privilege and oppression to become aware of and consider in terms of your own resilience as an LGBTQ person. The following resilience practice will help you further explore your religious/spiritual social identity.

RESILIENCE PRACTICE: Do You Have a Religious/Spiritual Identity?

The goal of this resilience practice is for you to discover whether a religious/spiritual identity is important to you and your resilience as an LGBTQ person. You may or may not have thought a lot about your religious/spiritual social identity. Or you may have an entirely different belief system or identity as agnostic or atheist. Answering the following questions should get you thinking about this part of you and its importance.

- Were you raised within a religious/spiritual community?

- Were you forced to go to a place of worship while growing up?

- Have you heard religious/spiritual people say anti-LGBTQ messages?

- Have you internalized anti-LGBTQ messages from religious/spiritual people?

- Have you heard positive messages about being LGBTQ and religious/spiritual?

- When you experience challenging times, do you engage in religious/spiritual practices?

As you read these questions, what came to mind? Write down those thoughts:

_____

_____

_____

_____

_____

Many thoughts may have come to mind for you as an LGBTQ person. You may realize you want to explore religious/spiritual traditions more—or less. You may realize you identify as atheist or agnostic. Whatever you realize, think about your experiences with and values of religious/spiritual traditions and how they may affect your resilience as an LGBTQ person. Remember, *you* get to decide what you do and do not believe—and those beliefs may change over time.

I was told that trans people do not have a lot of options when it comes to jobs.

—Anonymous

Social Class

Your access to financial resources has a great influence on your resilience as an LGBTQ person. Social class, also commonly called "socioeconomic status," refers to this access to resources. We just discussed the challenge of talking about race/ethnicity and exploring and valuing this part of yourself—well, the issue of social class can feel just as slippery. You may have grown up living in government-provided housing, but your family may have worked hard to not let this lack of financial resources show. You may have grown up in a family with plenty of financial resources, but your family may have worked hard to not let that abundance show. You may have grown up in a family where everything about social class was on the table and openly discussed, or it may have been reserved for adult conversation, so as a child you never heard people talk about social class.

All LGBTQ people receive messages about social class. And like other identities, social class can be fluid and change over time. A family's financial resources commonly increase and decrease, with periods of relative abundance and scarcity. Even in a family with plenty of financial resources, an adverse event—like divorce, death, a natural disaster, or a medical emergency—can quickly drain these resources. Or it can go the other way—perhaps your family had no financial resources, then all of a sudden you were attending private schools and getting a car for graduation.

However, because social class is such a taboo subject, many of us don't have the words to talk about it. Basically, having *enough* financial resources makes you middle class, *not enough* resources means you're poor or working class, and *more than enough* resources makes you upper class. Your social class, with its level of financial resources, can either buffer you from some of the anti-LGBTQ messages in society (having a computer or smartphone gives you access to positive LGBTQ messages, groups, and media) or make you more vulnerable (like becoming homeless if you're kicked out of your home for being LGBTQ, or struggling to find employment as an LGBTQ person). In the next resilience practice, you'll reflect on your experiences of social class as an LGBTQ person.

RESILIENCE PRACTICE: Social Class and LGBTQ Identities

The goal of this resilience practice is for you to explore your experiences of social class over time. Consider the following questions:

- What was the predominant social class you were raised in?

- Has your social class changed over your lifetime?

- When you realized you were LGBTQ, how did your social class influence you?

_____

_____

_____

_____

_____

What do your responses to these questions have to do with your resilience as an LGBTQ person? During times of greater social class privilege, were you able to be more protected from oppression as an LGBTQ person, such as having financial resources to seek out information or services, or being able to choose a livelihood in a more progressive and supportive work industry or geographic region? Or did it work the other way—where the more social class you had (like your family), the less resilient you felt as an LGBTQ person in terms of expressing your identity? How does your current social class increase or decrease your overall resilience as an LGBTQ person?

Intersectionality, *a concept I first heard in the 1990s from feminist women of color, refers to experiencing crosscutting discrimination and violence on the basis of one's different marginalized identities because of underlying conditions. Success for LGBT rights has to be measured not only as compartmentalized rights on the basis of sexual orientation, gender identity and gender expression, but in the context of the many common structures of domination that prevent equality.*

—Grace Poore, lesbian, South Asian American,
Indian-born filmmaker

Intersectionality: Further Valuing All of Who You Are

In the introduction, you learned about the importance of resilience in general and how it relates to being queer or trans; in this chapter you will explore a few discrete social identities that also influence your resilience. Although I discuss these identities separately, each of us is an *intersection* of all of these identities. At times it may feel as if some, such as gender and sexual orientation, intersect. Some of these intersections may seem to be in conflict. And some of these social identity intersections feel like they truly cannot be separated from one another. Mick Rehrig describes how he experiences the intersections of his identity related to his personal and professional life, and how these intersections help grow his resilience:

To be queer and trans and to be loved, fully, without apology or scorn; to build intentional and beloved community that witnesses and mirrors my own life, and expands its humanity in its differences (to paraphrase my partner). To work with queer and trans youth allows me to love my community, and subsequently, myself more. They help me to love, nurture, and forgive the kid I used to be, they help minimize and smash my internalized shame: my internalized oppression. They help me remember the privileges I have due to White supremacist capitalist patriarchy (to quote bell hooks) and to be of service in healing through affirmation, support, advocacy, and resistance. To continue to live, to love and allow myself to be loved, and to stand up and fight back.

—Mick Rehrig, White, trans man; parent, partner, and therapist

The next resilience practice will help you gauge your overall resilience across many of your social identities, by rating how important each is to you as a queer or trans person.

RESILIENCE PRACTICE: Rank Your Social Identities

The goal of this resilience practice is for you to understand how important each of your social identities is to your resilience in dealing with the challenges of being an LGBTQ person in society. Assign a ranking number to each one, with 1 to indicate the most important. You can assign the same ranking number to several identities if they seem to have equal value to you.

_____   Ability (emotional, physical, developmental)

_____   Age

_____   Geographic region

_____   Gender

_____   National origin

_____   Race/ethnicity

_____   Religion/spirituality/agnosticism/atheism

_____   Sexual orientation

_____   Social class

Now read back through your rankings. Which identities are most important to you? Which did you rank lower? What overlaps do you notice among the rankings? Were certain identities tougher to rank? How might these identities relate to your experiences of privilege and oppression? This exercise is important because there may be identities that you have yet to experience pride in that are crucial components of your resilience as an LGBTQ person. There may be experiences of privilege—like race/ethnicity or social class—that can help you combat the effects of LGBTQ oppression, and there may be experiences of oppression that increase the threats to your resilience.

When it comes to my own intersections of identity, I too have trouble knowing how to separate my gender, sexual orientation, racial/ethnic, and religious/spiritual social identities. I just *know* what it feels like to be a queer, multiracial, South Asian, Sikh, nonbinary person. When I pay attention to privilege and oppression, things start to become more clear. For example, I would further describe my identities related to privilege:

I am a queer, multiracial, South Asian, Sikh woman with class, educational, and U.S.-born citizen privilege who is temporarily able-bodied.

When I then start to reflect on how my resilience is informed by the intersections of these identities, the description of my identities shifts:

I am a queer, multiracial, South Asian Sikh woman with class, educational, and U.S.-born citizen privilege who is temporarily able-bodied. The pride I have as a Sikh helps me bounce back from hard times as an LGBTQ person, because my religious/spiritual values include the importance of truth, justice, and serving community. My connections with multiracial mentors and young people in my life help me remember the beauty in being of mixed racial heritage, and I am embedded with a queer and trans

South Asian community with whom I can share my love of South Asian food, dance, and cultural values. My educational privilege has helped me attain more class privilege, and I use these two privileges and my U.S.-born citizen privilege to advocate for others. Advocating for others is also a part of my religious/spiritual heritage and upbringing, so all of these experiences of privilege and oppression are intersectional for me.

The following resilience practice will help you look more deeply into your intersections of identity with privilege, oppression, and overall intersectional resilience.

RESILIENCE PRACTICE: Your Intersectional Resilience Related to Privilege and Oppression

The aim of this resilience practice is to build on your rankings in the previous resilience practice and connect these important identity intersections to your experiences of privilege and oppression as I just shared in my example. Consider the following questions, then respond:

- What are the important intersections of your identities as an LGBTQ person?

- How do these intersections relate to privilege and oppression?

- How do these intersections make you more resilient as an LGBTQ person?

_____

_____

_____

_____

_____

_____

What did you notice about your intersectional resilience? Were they different from your resilience related to your single identities, like race/ethnicity, disability, and social class? How does your privilege help buffer you from discrimination as a queer or trans person—and how do identities related to oppression influence your resilience when you consider them all together?

Resilience Wrap-Up

Queer and trans people have so many more social identities that are important to us than just being LGBTQ. Reflecting on which of these social identities are more or less important to you helps you become more resilient to challenges you face as an LGBTQ person, because you have the opportunity to develop pride and confidence in these identities, which in turn increases your resilience. Keep developing your resilience as an LGBTQ person with multiple identities through:

- Learning more about your social identities in addition to being LGBTQ

- Connecting with people (LGBTQ and cisgender) who share a social identity with you

- Exploring what you like and do not like about a social identity

- Identifying positive and negative messages you have heard about your social identities

- Considering how you might have internalized negative messages about certain social identities, and challenging these beliefs

- Realizing that a mixture of privilege and oppression experiences can influence your resilience

- Embracing the intersections of your unique LGBTQ identities with other social identities

Now that you have explored your resilience related to your multiple identities as a queer and trans person, in Chapter 3 you will delve further into identifying how you have internalized negative messages about being LGBTQ and learn how to externalize them.

Further Identifying Negative Messages

Resilience is all about bouncing back from adversity, and that means making sure you know what you are bouncing back *from* so you can better take care of yourself. You explored some of these adversities in previous chapters. In this chapter you'll take a internal inventory to pinpoint the specific negative messages you've been given about your sexual orientation, your gender, and other salient aspects of your identity. This deeper look can help you develop skills to name, externalize, and challenge these negative messages.

Sources of Negative Messages

Before you think about the sources of the negative messages you've received about who you are, I encourage you to revisit the discussion of minority stress in the introduction. Part of this stress is from microaggressions—those everyday insensitive or insulting remarks that queer and trans people experience in their interpersonal relationships within their families, workplaces, schools, and other community environments. These indignities may be intended or unintended, but either way, it's hard to know what to say, think, or do in response.

For example, you might be in a school or work setting and hear someone say, "That person acted *so gay.*" Bisexual people may hear, "One day, you will meet the *right* person"; trans people may hear, "It must be frustrating to know you will never be a *real* woman." Because microaggressions are everyday indignities, they can happen in many different situations related to common events (such as holidays or weddings), ways of interacting (like attempts at humor or support), and daily living (for example, when taking public transportation or going to the movies). Remember that the discriminatory content in microaggressions can range from overt to covert. Here are some other examples of microaggressive statements queer and trans people might hear:

From family:

- "Do you have to bring your partner for your visit next month?"

- "Growing up, I always thought you might turn out gay."

- "I knew I should not have let you play with dolls growing up."

- "Jill and Rasheeda can fly from New York to Idaho for the holidays, because they don't have kids."

From friends:

- "I am so glad you told me you are trans! You are the first trans person I know!"

- "It must be so hard to be a girl after 5:00 p.m. when your five o'clock shadow starts to show."

- "Are you sure you are not just a butch lesbian?"

- "This is my best friend who is gay."

From work or school colleagues:

- "It must be so hard to be gay."

- "I would never have known you were not a woman!"

- "Does being bisexual make your partner worry?"

- "If you and your partners are lesbians, who plays the role of the 'man'?"

From public spaces:

- "Who is the woman in your relationship?"

- "I have a friend who is just like you."

- "If you are gay, shouldn't you be in a different locker room?"

- "You must be in the wrong restroom."

As you read this sample list of microaggressive statements, notice how you feel. Were there some that were more subtle, so it was difficult to figure out why the statements or questions were discriminatory? Did you find yourself nodding your head in agreement with some of the statements and questions? Did you notice you had a more intense reaction reading the microaggressions in one particular category?

RESILIENCE PRACTICE: Identifying My Personal Experiences of Microaggressions

Now it's time to zero in on your personal experience. Take a moment to list some of the specific microaggressive statements you've heard.

From Family:

Microaggression 1: _____

_____

Microaggression 2: _____

_____

Microaggression 3: _____

_____

Microaggression 4: _____

_____

From Friends:

Microaggression 1: _____

_____

Microaggression 2: _____

_____

Microaggression 3: _____

_____

Microaggression 4: _____

_____

From Work or School Colleagues:

Microaggression 1: _____

_____

Microaggression 2: _____

_____

Microaggression 3: _____

_____

Microaggression 4: _____

_____

From Public Spaces:

Microaggression 1: _____

_____

Microaggression 2: _____

_____

Microaggression 3: _____

_____

Microaggression 4: _____

_____

Now check in with how you felt as you listed these personal experiences of microaggressions. Did your heart start to race? Did you begin to feel sad, fearful, or angry? Or maybe you felt happy or even proud that you know how to respond to some of the microaggressions you hear. Any and all feelings you have are valid.

Responses to Negative Messages

Now, let's talk about the next step of becoming more resilient to microaggressions: understanding your specific responses. As an LGBTQ person, when you hear these negative messages often you can experience shock. For example, you might think, "Did they *really* just say that to me?" Then it becomes very real that it *was* said and that it was not OK for you to hear. Still, you may experience doubt and confusion, leading to self-questioning; for example:

- Did they maybe not mean what they just said?

- Am I just being a "too sensitive" lesbian right now?

- What am I doing to make it OK for them to say this to me as a gay person?

- They must be trying their best right now to use my pronouns; why should I get angry?

- How can I get them to stop saying those biphobic things to me?

- If I were better at _____ [fill in the blank], I could probably respond to them better.

- If I say something, it is going to make it worse.

- Why does this keep happening to me? Maybe I am asking for it.

In the following resilience practice, you can identify your own examples from your experiences responding to microaggressions.

RESILIENCE PRACTICE: Identifying Your Common Thoughts in Response to Microaggressions

Of course, each person's experience is different. This practice will help you zero in on your own responses. When you read the preceding examples, did other questions or thoughts that come to mind that you have experienced? Write them here:

_____

_____

_____

_____

How did it feel to gain more insight about your common internal reactions to microaggressions? Were you able to identify the self-questioning that microaggressions can provoke within you? This self-questioning makes complete sense, as the shock of experiencing a microaggression makes it hard to digest in the moment what just happened. This shock and self-questioning also stops you from responding to the person in the moment, and then you may beat yourself up afterward thinking about what you should have said. Or you may think you overreacted and that you are at fault for your feelings. Microaggressions are truly *crazy-making* experiences, because you are in fact hearing things that are not OK—and then you question yourself.

Emma Blackwell developed resilience through acknowledging the challenges she faced, and then externalizing anti-trans messages.

Being trans isn't always hard. There are such beautiful and amazing times being trans, but those times when things do seem too tough or even insurmountable, I found a few things that simply made it better for me. I often would reflect on all the times I hid my true self, and there was so much of that, and then I look at all the relief and self-happiness I have found since coming out. It's so hard to beat that sense of overwhelming personal happiness and contentment. For me, it has always been important to stand up and be counted, so I find strength in becoming more and more active and fighting for all of us. It is such an empowering experience, whether I work alone in the fight or, even better, when I join with others for the cause. We are awesome, and I find such strength in working toward a better future.

—Emma Blackwell, White, trans woman, activist

Being Prepared to Respond to Microaggressions

It's difficult to hold people accountable for microaggressions because they are often interacting with others based on heteronormative attitudes (prioritizing straight and heterosexual people) that are unconsciously embedded into everyday life interactions, like assuming everyone is straight. Still, experiencing ongoing microaggressions and responding to them is an exhausting process. This exhaustion is real, and the hurt can be internalized and build up over time so that you become numb to experiences that should not be happening to you.

This exhaustion and numbness make it clear why it's important to be prepared to respond. Sometimes this response is external—saying or doing something so you do not walk away from the experience feeling bad about your response (or lack of response). Other times the response should be internal, reminding yourself of your worth and value as a queer or trans person. If you have ever received fire safety training, you'll know that firefighters talk a lot about emergency preparedness. Firefighters drive home these emergency preparedness messages to the point that you have internalized the important steps you should take next, such as "Stop, drop, and roll!" You can establish your own three steps to enhance your resilience to microaggressions: "Name, validate, and act!" First, you name what is happening. Second, you validate any feelings you have. Third, you decide whether an action is needed in that moment. Let's break down these three steps a little further.

Name Microaggressions When They Happen

The first step, naming, could also be called the "I am not crazy—that *did* just happen" step. Naming means that you learn to recognize that a microaggression is happening. Often, microaggressions are so insidious that you get used to them, and you're socialized to ignore them. Naming entails acknowledging to yourself that what you heard or experienced was not in alignment with your self-worth as a queer or trans person—or worse, it was anti-LGBTQ.

Here's an example. Say you identify as a trans woman, and you date women. One day when you're at work, in a group conversation you mention that you went on a date to a movie but you alone enjoyed it, and someone says, "You should let your boyfriend choose the movie next time." Naming means that you as a queer or lesbian trans woman know that a microaggression just happened, because heteronormative assumptions about whom you would date were embedded in this person's question. This step is important because of the everyday nature of microaggressions, and it can create some of the following internal responses, depending on the microaggression:

- I just heard a microaggression.

- I just experienced a microaggression.

- I want to question myself now, but that was indeed a discriminatory remark.

- I was just treated poorly because I am queer or trans.

- That statement was anti-queer and anti-trans.

- This person would not have said this to someone who was cisgender or straight.

Naming a microaggression gives you a chance to acknowledge the situation that you are experiencing, so you can be more resilient and protect yourself.

Validate Your Feelings

Once you have named that a microaggression has happened, the second step is to validate how you are feeling. Because microaggressions can happen quickly and catch us off guard, the previous step of naming that it happened can help you slow down and ask yourself, "How do I feel about this statement or behavior?" It is natural to have a wide range of emotional responses, from anger to sadness to fear. Numbness, as I have discussed, is also a common reaction, but it is still a feeling that gives you some information on your emotional state. Slowing down to validate your feelings acknowledges that those feelings are legitimate data that help guide your decision-making and actions. Here are some other common feelings that might come up for you within the larger categories of anger, fear, sadness, and numbness:

- **Anger:** frustrated, aggressive, exasperated, disgusted, enraged

- **Fear:** embarrassed, nervous, suspicious, frightened, terrified

- **Sadness:** lonely, ashamed, depressed, hurt, disappointed

- **Numbness:** disbelieving, withdrawn, shocked, indifferent

When you have identified the feelings you have as a result of the microaggression (naming), you can validate them; for example:

"Because I just experienced _____ [naming the microaggression], it makes sense that I would feel _____ [validating the emotion]."

You may very well have more than one feeling come up in response to a microaggression (like feeling disappointed *and* scared), or you may have one feeling that is quickly replaced by another (like feeling angry and then feeling sad). Make sure you validate *all* of the feelings that come up for you.

Act

After you have named the microaggression and validated your emotional response, it is time to act. Acting means that you *act* to protect yourself, so acting can entail either an internal action or an external action, or it may include both.

INTERNAL ACTIONS

Internal actions include possible thoughts or affirmations that reflect your value as an LGBTQ person; for example:

- Thinking, "I am valuable as a queer or trans person."

- Affirming to yourself, "I do not deserve this treatment as a queer or trans person."

- Acknowledging to yourself, "I deserve to be treated respectfully and with dignity as a queer or trans person."

EXTERNAL ACTIONS

An external action might include saying something to the person who committed the microaggression, such as the following.

Verbal Actions:

- When you said _____, that wasn't affirming of who I am as a queer or trans person.

- When you said _____, you assumed _____ about me as a queer or trans person.

- When you said _____, I felt excluded as a queer or trans person.

- When you said _____, I felt _____ as a queer or trans person.

- You may not have realized it, but when you said _____, you weren't supportive of me as a queer or trans person.

- Please don't say _____ to me again.

External action can also include engaging in a short-term or long-term protective behavior in response to the microaggression. Like verbal actions, behavioral actions can entail a variety of responses.

Behavioral Actions:

- Removing yourself from the situation

- Seeking a safe space

- Connecting with social support

- Engaging in self-care activities, such as practicing mindfulness, reading, or taking a bath

- Journaling or blogging about your experience

- Attending a support group or counseling

Practice New Responses to Microaggressions

Developing the skills of naming, validating, and acting in response to microaggressions takes some practice. As you learned in the introduction, developing resilience is like building muscle. Working on the discrete aspects of resilience over time, with lots of practice, strengthens that muscle and gives you the strength you need to challenge oppression and embrace your self-worth. Let's read through a few case scenarios to see what the three steps of naming, validating, and acting in response to microaggressions might look like all together.

GENDER MICROAGGRESSION

Scenario One. A White trans woman, Geena, is taking the subway to work. As she enters the train and sits in the available seat, her fellow passenger says, "You look just like a woman—how long have you been on hormones?"

Naming: Geena says to herself, "That was not an OK thing to say, and I may not be safe here."

Validating: Geena acknowledges her emotions of anger and fear.

Acting: Geena reminds herself internally that her medical chart is private, and that she gets to define her own womanhood for herself. She moves to another seat on the train, and she calls her friend to share what happened.

Scenario Two. A Latinx, lesbian woman, Daria, is getting coffee at work. Her coworker friend from a different floor sees her for the first time in a month and exclaims, "You are looking more feminine—I like this look!"

Naming: Daria says to herself, "I just heard a microaggression."

Validating: Daria pauses to check in with her feelings, and she identifies feeling indifferent at first, but then uncomfortable with her coworker.

Acting: Daria tells her coworker, "You may not have realized it, but when you said I looked more 'feminine,' I felt uncomfortable with what you said."

SEXUAL ORIENTATION MICROAGGRESSION

Scenario One. A Native American, gay man, Jared, is walking into his daughter's school. Another father is picking up his child, and he says to Jared, "What are you and your wife doing for the weekend?"

Naming: Jared says to himself, "He probably doesn't realize it, but he just made a lot of assumptions about who I am—that is a microaggression."

Validating: Jared checks in with his feelings and notices he feels withdrawn, and doesn't feel like "making a fuss" about this father's mistake.

Acting: Jared internally tells himself, "Being a gay father is something to be proud of, and I can decide whether to address this or not with this fellow dad." Jared decides not to address the microaggression, but does speak to the principal about having an LGBTQ training at the next PTA meeting.

Scenario Two. A Filipino-American, bisexual boy, Crisanto, is a junior at his high school. His teacher asks him which girl he wants to ask to the prom.

Naming: Crisanto says to himself, "My teacher just said a microaggression, assuming I am straight."

Validating: Crisanto takes an inventory of his feelings. He feels angry.

Acting: Crisanto internally tells himself, "People do not know a lot about being bisexual. I don't have to come out to this teacher, but I can if I want to." Crisanto decides to tell his teacher, "I appreciate you asking the question, but you assumed I am straight—and that is a big assumption about people. I actually am bisexual, and right now I am dating boys—but I haven't decided whom I will bring."

As you read the case scenarios, did you notice that the people really varied in what they decided to do or not do? The naming and validating steps were consistent across the scenarios (though with varying emotions), but the acting steps resulted in different decisions. Some were motivated by safety, others by current relationships or the setting in which the microaggression occurred. Regardless of the different decision made in the acting step, each action shared the common theme of the queer or trans person deciding for themselves what was in their best interest. See the next resilience practice to further explore microaggressions.

RESILIENCE PRACTICE: How Do Microaggressions Relate to My Life as an LGBTQ Person?

In this practice, you'll write your own case scenarios related to your gender and sexual orientation—or any other identity, such as race/ethnicity or social class—using real-life situations in which you have experienced microaggressions.

Microaggression: _____

_____

Naming: _____

_____

Validating: _____

_____

Acting: _____

_____

Microaggression: _____

_____

Naming: _____

_____

Validating: _____

_____

Acting: _____

_____

Do you feel your resilience muscle growing after writing your own scenarios? The more you prepare for your responses to microaggressions and remind yourself that you get to decide what actions to take, the more the self-questioning related to these negative messages will decrease and the more your resilience muscle develops! At http://www.newharbinger.com/39461, you can download a worksheet version of this exercise to keep your resilience muscle growing.

I am no longer accepting the things I cannot change. I am changing the things I cannot accept.

—Angela Davis, Black, cisgender, professor
and activist

Beyond Microaggressions: Externalizing Anti-LGBTQ Messages

It's important to develop skills to be prepared for microaggressions so you can move through those experiences with minimal impact on your self-esteem and self-confidence as a queer or trans person, further building your resilience. Simultaneously, you can learn to intentionally externalize negative messages you hear about yourself. Some of these messages are connected to myths about queer and trans people, such as that being queer or trans is a choice. Other negative messages have to do with a lack of knowledge, such as about queer and trans historical figures and role models (like Audre Lorde, Bayard Rustin, Christine Jorgensen, Harvey Milk) in our school textbooks and college courses. We have discussed some of these negative messages and myths in previous chapters; now we'll explore the internalization processes.

Internalized oppression refers to negative societal attitudes about a group without privilege in society that a person internalizes and starts to believe about themselves or others in their group. So, internalized oppression is comprised of these negative beliefs you have taken to heart and unintentionally made a part of your own belief system. You may be thinking this is not a problem for you: "Well, my life is not so bad. I know queer and trans people deserve to be treated well. I don't have any negative ideas about my community." But internalization is hard to avoid, given the pervasive oppressive messages and microaggressions in society. And this can be a serious threat to your resilience as an LGBTQ person. Believe me, I am tempted to think about that as well. However, anti-LGBTQ oppression is so pervasive not only as overt oppression, but also more insidiously as covert and overt acts of omission.

Here's how Lauren Lukkarila, a queer, gender-transgressive person, transformed these messages into reminders of her own unique resilience:

> "You're different in a different way." Hearing these words from the mouth of an elder family member I loved dearly scared me—even as an adult. But these words also excited me on some level because they acknowledged that I had been seen—really seen—despite the lifetime I spent disciplining myself to "not show myself." My resilience as child and young person was the basic survival kind—know your enemy and be invisible to the best of your ability. I still feel that urge in me even now, but now I know people who have chosen other forms of resilience. I've seen them choose to thrive and not just survive, and I've seen that there's a community of folks—and it's bigger than I would ever have thought—that support thriving.
>
> —Lauren Lukkarila

Even if you reach a place where you believe there is nothing wrong with being queer or trans, your quest for resilience entails asking yourself what you learned that was awesome about being queer or trans. The following resilience practice invites you to explore some of the messages you have heard as an LGBTQ person.

RESILIENCE PRACTICE: LGBTQ Messages—What Have You "Heard"?

The purpose of this resilience practice is to really dig in and identify the types of LGBTQ-affirming messages you have heard. Consider the following questions and explore them in the space provided:

When you were growing up, what positive messages did you hear about queer and trans people?

_____

_____

What positive stories did you hear from school teachers about queer and trans people?

_____

_____

Who were the queer and trans leaders you heard about, across race/ethnicity, gender, class, disability, and country, among other identities?

_____

_____

What positive messages about your sexuality did you learn in your family, school, religious/spiritual institutions, and other community centers?

_____

_____

What positive messages did you hear about queer and trans people from cisgender and straight people?

_____

_____

While growing up, what positive queer and trans events were you exposed to or taken to?

_____

_____

While growing up, what sex-positive messages did you hear about queer and trans people?

_____

_____

It is my greatest hope and goal that eventually you will live in a society where these questions become obsolete, in the sense that queer and trans people are valued and integrated into all aspects of society and institutions of all sorts. Until that happens, it is vital that you are intentional in healing wounds related not only to overt anti-LGBTQ oppression, but also to the withholding of your queer and trans histories and positive messages of affirmation across your life span.

RESILIENCE PRACTICE: What Have You Been Taught to Believe?

In this practice, you'll explore the negative messages you've received about being queer or trans. Write the anti-LGBTQ messages you heard growing up:

_____

_____

_____

_____

_____

What do you notice about the anti-LGBTQ messages you learned growing up? Did you receive more overt (obvious) messages or more covert (masked, hidden, "coded") messages?

RESILIENCE PRACTICE: What Do You Want to Believe about Being Queer or Trans?

Now take some time to consider positive messages about being queer or trans that you wish you had heard or that you think you should have heard while growing up, and write them here:

_____

_____

_____

_____

_____

_____

How did it feel to list positive messages you *should* have received about being queer or trans after assembling the previous list of negative LGBTQ messages? Part of resilience is knowing not only the anti-LGBTQ messages that are bad for your mental health, but also the positive LGBTQ messages that address the gaps in your learning about being LGBTQ. Read this list of positive messages about being LGBTQ and see whether there is any overlap with the list you just made:

- LGBTQ people are important and valuable members of society.

- Queer and trans people have been positive contributors to society throughout history.

- LGBTQ people have existed on every continent and in every culture around the world. In many cultures, queer and trans people were considered sacred and participated in important cultural and spiritual rituals.

- There have been important queer and trans liberation movements across the world, as LGBTQ people have fought for their rights and against discrimination. Cisgender and straight people have supported LGBTQ people in these liberation movements.

- Queer and trans people deserve to be treated well in society.

- LGBTQ people should be treated with respect and dignity at school and work.

- Queer and trans people can be strong leaders.

- LGBTQ people can make important contributions to society.

- Queer and trans rights should be protected in society.

What differences can you see between this LGBTQ-positive list and the list you made about what you should have heard growing up about LGBTQ people? How do you feel noticing these differences?

Internalizing Positive Messages about LGBTQ People

Now that you have explored how to move through microaggressions and embrace your dignity as a queer or trans person, and you've identified both negative and positive LGBTQ messages, let's talk about specific strategies for internalizing positive messages about queer and trans people.

You can think about this internalization as a personal reeducation. Think about it. What if you were raised by your family, school, and community to believe that the earth is flat? Wouldn't that be a sad and sorry state of affairs, to walk around believing something that is not true? Wouldn't you desperately want to tell someone who believed that the world was flat that it actually was round? Well, that is exactly what this reeducation is about—it is about making sure you know the best of your history as a queer or trans person. It is about taking a journey to learn more about the dynamic brilliance and creativity that has existed within the queer and trans community for hundreds of years, so that you can know more about yourself as a queer or trans person and how your life is a continuation of this legacy.

Education either functions as an instrument which is used to facilitate the integration of the younger generation into the logic of the present system and bring about conformity, or it becomes the practice of freedom, the means by which [people] deal critically and creatively with reality and discover how to participate in the transformation of their world.

—Paulo Freire, Brazilian educator and author

There are many ways to learn about queer and trans history—including books, websites, and museum exhibits, as well as directly from those who have lived it. So where do you get started in learning about the history of your community? For instance, did you know that the "architect" of Dr. Martin Luther King's 1963 March on Washington (where he delivered the famous "I Have a Dream" speech) was Bayard Rustin, a gay African American man? Did you know that Rustin was also the person who introduced Gandhi's nonviolent civil disobedience to Dr. King? This is a crucial aspect of LGBTQ history you should have been taught in school!

Read through the Resources section at the end of this workbook to find ways to learn more about the history of your queer and trans community.

Learning about queer and trans history can help you not only learn more about the history of your people across cultural groups but also develop pride in the accomplishments of your community and knowledge about how LGBTQ people have stood up against anti-queer and anti-trans oppression over time. As you develop this pride you can also develop strong self-esteem and confidence about being LGBTQ yourself. You will explore self-esteem and pride further in Chapter 4.

Resilience Wrap-Up

When you, as an LGBTQ person, can recognize oppression when it occurs and can identify negative and positive messages related to being LGBTQ, you can increase your resilience by knowing the steps to take after a microaggression. Knowing your queer and trans history strengthens your LGBTQ pride, as you realize you are the next generation of a vibrant and amazing community. When you need to counter negative LGBTQ messages, remember the following:

- Remember that microaggressions can occur with family and friends, as well as in public spaces.

- Take the three steps to enhance your resilience: name, validate, and act.

- Prepare for situations where you are likely to experience microaggressions by thinking through them in advance.

- Realize that *you* get to decide how you respond to microaggressions: sometimes a response is needed in the moment, other times not.

- Identify areas for healing by reflecting on what you have been taught to believe about yourself as a queer and trans person.

- Strengthen your resilience by identifying positive messages you *should* have heard growing up as an LGBTQ person.

- Get to know LGBTQ history, to contextualize your life as a queer and trans person, learn more about your community, and develop LGBTQ pride.

Being prepared and knowing how to address microaggressions increases your resilience as an LGBTQ person. In Chapter 4, you'll explore how to develop the resilience strategy of knowing your self-worth and valuing yourself.

CHAPTER 4

Knowing Your Self-Worth

Because schools seldom teach LGBTQ history, much less the value of queer and trans people in society, educating yourself about your own self-worth is an important aspect of building your resilience. Self-worth refers to the degree of value and importance you place on living your life. LGBTQ people have higher rates of depression, suicidality, self-injury, substance abuse, and other mental health challenges than the general population (Institute of Medicine, 2011). Why are queer and trans people subject to these increased risks? Is it because queer and trans people are inherently more flawed than cisgender and straight people? The answer is an emphatic "No!" However, when negative messages about an LGBTQ person's self and community are so prevalent in society, these thoughts can become internalized, as discussed in Chapter 3. Then you start to believe these thoughts and subsequently feel like there is something inherently wrong with you. Although your rational mind may be able to tell you that this is simply not true, you may still *feel* this way.

Building resilience includes assessing your sense of self-worth and self-esteem. In this chapter, you will explore how much you value yourself as a queer or trans person and how you can develop a greater sense of self-worth. In doing so, you will reflect on your self-esteem as an LGBTQ person, and how you can develop assertiveness skills with others and also challenge the voice of your inner critic—which all of us have.

Over the years, I've learned to embrace both my love of lipstick and my facial hair, my affinity for sequins and my broad shoulders.

—Anonymous

Understanding Self-Esteem

When people talk about self-worth, self-esteem is a large part of that construct. Self-worth refers to how much you value yourself, whereas self-esteem can be a practical reflection of your self-worth. Much of the research on self-esteem in the average population examines self-esteem as confidence in one's own abilities. Self-efficacy is another word for this idea, which refers to your belief in your own ability to do things well. Alberto Perez developed a strong sense of self-esteem and resilience from the support he received from his family:

Before I became a teenager, I realized I was gay. I really didn't experience trauma, because I felt that being gay was an easy thing to accept about myself. I never really felt that I wasn't accepted, because my family was very accepting and loving to one another. It was more difficult as I was coming out and accepting who I truly was when I got older. Even though I had the support of my family, I did still experience some type of fear that I wouldn't be accepted. Today, I accept myself, and I know that the family I was raised in and my work environment were very accepting. I make sure to surround myself with loving people and positive people, and this is a conscious choice for me as a gay man. I know my family laid a loving support for me, and that made all of the difference with my resilience.

—Alberto Perez, Latinx, cisgender, gay man

Each of us has our own journey in finding our self-esteem. This journey can be affected by many factors, such as:

- Negative messages from family, friends, school, work, and other institutions

- Experiences of emotional, physical, sexual, spiritual, or other types of abuse

- Unstable home environments, such as lacking financial resources or experiencing divorce in the family

- Negative life events, such as losing a job, moving, or changing schools

- Discrimination

You can see that everything on this list could potentially influence one's self-esteem. I say potentially, because your resilience does help you counter these life experiences. However, if you have experienced multiple factors like these, it may be more challenging to learn to value yourself. Additionally, no matter where you are with your self-esteem related to these factors, the last one—discrimination—can turn your entire life upside down. For instance, you may feel really good about who you are and your ability to engage in various activities. Then an anti-LGBTQ situation arises (such as being called a "fag" or a "sinner"), and you may suddenly feel vulnerable and question yourself. So no matter how your self-esteem has fluctuated in the course of your life, having a plan to build your self-esteem as a queer or trans person will help you be more resilient in all areas of your life.

I have had to face a lot of internalized homophobia and ableism. As someone who lives with bipolar, and is queer and a woman, I have often felt crazy and like a nuisance to culture. I didn't feel valuable. It wasn't until I started working within the queer community, and raising the voices of queer disabled women, that I began to challenge the oppression within myself. Through the support of mentors and peers, I became confident enough to challenge my internal oppression—whether sexism, homophobia, or ableism—and build resilience. Knowing my own emotions and identities, and being able to accept them, has helped me feel more in control of myself and feel powerful.

—Nat Truszczynski, White, queer, cisgender woman

To most effectively build your self-esteem, it's helpful to have a sense of the factors that have influenced your current self-esteem. So take some time now to identify those factors with the next resilience practice.

RESILIENCE PRACTICE: Identifying Factors That Have Influenced Your Self-Esteem

Read through the following items and think about how these may have affected you through the years. Write down your reflections after each one.

Negative messages from family, friends, school, work, and other institutions

_____

_____

_____

_____

Experiences of emotional, physical, sexual, spiritual, or other types of abuse

_____

_____

_____

_____

Unstable home environments, like lacking financial resources or experiencing a divorce in the family

_____

_____

_____

_____

Negative life events, such as losing a job, moving, or changing schools

_____

_____

_____

_____

As you completed this practice, did you notice that certain factors had a greater negative influence than others on your self-esteem as a queer or trans person?

Next, let's explore some potential positive influences on your self-esteem. Again, read through them, think how they may have affected you, then write down your reflections.

Positive messages from family, friends, school, work, and other institutions

_____

_____

_____

_____

Experiences of empowerment

_____

_____

_____

_____

Stable home environments

_____

_____

_____

_____

Other positive life events

_____

_____

_____

_____

As you wrote about the negative and positive influences on your self-esteem, which of these do you think had the most impact on you as an LGBTQ person? When you think about your self-esteem as a queer or trans person, have you had more negative influences, more positive influences, or about the same of both negative and positive? Keep these in mind as you complete a more general measure of self-esteem in the next resilience practice.

RESILIENCE PRACTICE: The Rosenberg Self-Esteem Scale (1965): Taking a Pulse of Your General Self-Esteem

Let's assess your general self-esteem before you explore self-esteem specific to being LGBTQ. The Rosenberg Self-Esteem Scale (1965) has been used for over fifty years to measure self-esteem; with it, you can easily get an idea of what your current self-esteem is.

Read the following list of statements concerning your general feelings about yourself.

If you strongly agree with the statement, circle SA.

If you agree, circle A.

If you disagree, circle D.

If you strongly disagree, circle SD.

My Feelings about Myself	Strongly Agree	Agree	Disagree	Strongly Disagree
1. I feel that I'm a person of worth, at least on an equal plane with others.	SA	A	D	SD
2. I feel that I have a number of good qualities.	SA	A	D	SD
3. All in all, I am inclined to feel that I am a failure.	SA	A	D	SD
4. I am able to do things as well as most other people.	SA	A	D	SD
5. I feel I do not have much to be proud of.	SA	A	D	SD
6. I take a positive attitude toward myself.	SA	A	D	SD
7. On the whole, I am satisfied with myself.	SA	A	D	SD
8. I wish I could have more respect for myself.	SA	A	D	SD
9. I certainly feel useless at times.	SA	A	D	SD
10. At times I think I am no good at all.	SA	A	D	SD

Score your answers as follows:

For items 1, 2, 4, 6, and 7:

Strongly agree = 3

Agree = 2

Disagree = 1

Strongly Disagree = 0

For items 3, 5, 8, 9, and 10 (which are reversed in score):

Strongly agree = 0

Agree = 1

Disagree = 2

Strongly Disagree = 3

Your Self-Esteem Score = _____.

The scale ranges from 0 to 30. Scores over 25 suggest high self-esteem; scores between 15 and 25 are within the average range; scores below 15 suggest low self-esteem.

Was your self-esteem score in the low, average, or high range? No matter what your score is, is it a surprise to you? Also, keep in mind that you are scoring yourself on this self-esteem scale to collect some data to begin exploring, with the ultimate goal of *strengthening your self-esteem.*

Next, respond to the following questions to reflect on your self-esteem score further and identify the areas to work on in developing your resilience.

What strengths do you think you have when it comes to your self-esteem?

_____

_____

_____

_____

What would you like to improve when it comes to your self-esteem?

_____

_____

_____

_____

What have you been told about your self-esteem?

_____

_____

_____

_____

What would you like to be able to say about your self-esteem?

_____

_____

_____

_____

As you reflected more deeply on your self-esteem score, was it easy or hard to identify your strengths and areas to improve with your self-esteem? Do you feel pretty good about your self-esteem, or do you want to increase it and maybe do not know how to do so? Hold on to these thoughts as you next explore your self-esteem as a queer or trans person and the different dimensions of self-esteem that you can work on to build your resilience. (If at any point you'd like to complete the assessment again, download the worksheet version of this exercise available at http://www.newharbinger.com/39461.)

Nurturing Queer and Trans Self-Esteem

What does self-esteem that's specific to queer and trans people look like? This question brings us back to the internalization of negative LGBTQ messages. This internalization can feed that critical inner voice that picks apart everything you do. This internalization can also decrease our motivation to be ourselves. When you don't believe that being LGBTQ is one of the best things about you, then you have a hard time going after your dreams and/or feeling that a happy life is possible for you. As you read through the rest of this chapter, you will learn different aspects of nurturing your self-esteem: challenging your inner critic, identifying thoughts that make you feel good, being assertive, and venturing outside of your comfort zone.

The fact is, I'm gay, always have been, always will be, and I couldn't be any more happy, comfortable with myself, and proud.

—Anderson Cooper, White, cisgender, gay man

Revising Your Internal Critic

A big self-esteem killer is often your very own self. When you internalize ideas that you are not worthy and begin to believe you have little or no value, you become very skilled at generating thoughts that keep you validating this low self-esteem. We all have an inner critic; it's that voice that pretty much tells you that you are doing everything, most things, or some things wrong. The life factors I discussed earlier in this chapter can affect the degree to which you believe that you are not worthy or capable.

It is helpful to start to get to know this inner critic—and possibly even give him/her/them/zir a name. Why a name? Recall Chapter 3, where I talked about the three-step process of naming, validating, and acting. Naming is a powerful act. Naming tells you that something is *real*. Therefore, giving your inner critic a name can acknowledge this part of you so you can start to develop a relationship with it.

I have named my inner critic Gertrude. Gertrude has a lot to say about everything I do. She has even been present as I write this workbook. Gertrude, as my innermost and most vociferous critic, tells me, "Well, what's the point of writing this book?" and "Who is going to read it anyway?" You can tell that Gertrude is the enemy of my self-esteem. In fact, her goal is to knock me down and make sure that I do not succeed in life. Here are some things she has to say to me:

- You can't do it.

- Why even try?

- Don't you realize what they will think of you?

- You will do a horrible job.

- You will mess this up.

- Remember the last time you got this wrong?

- You will never be as good as _____ (fill in the blank).

Gertrude has some harsh things to say, right? But here is the strange and very important thing about Gertrude. I have made it a point over the years to love and welcome her. She sits on my shoulder and squawks in my ear. Now that I know she exists, I can tell her, "Yeah, yeah. I hear you. And I am so sorry you feel that way." When I acknowledge that my inner critic voice is there, something even stranger happens. Gertrude starts to settle down and move out of my way. I like to think that once I acknowledge her concerns, she heads to the mall to do some shopping. She for sure will be right back and have more to say. But Gertrude no longer has the same sort of power she once had over me.

Everyone has some version of an inner Gertrude—a gremlin voice that wants to tear you down, beat you up, and make sure you fail. Why? Because our inner critic actually is deathly afraid of getting hurt, being rejected, and never being a success, it likes to plays it safe by keeping us "in line." The trouble is, society has already been playing a doozy on us through criticism, shame, betrayal, denigration, disapproval—you get the drift. So, making friends with your inner gremlin and getting to know how this little critic ticks is an important aspect of growing your self-esteem. To explore your inner critic further, complete the next resilience practice.

RESILIENCE PRACTICE: Getting to Know Our Inner Critic and Gremlin

Let's explore what your inner critic and gremlin sounds like for you. Consider the following questions and then write your response.

Who is your inner critic and gremlin?

_____

What kinds of things does this part of you say to get in the way of your feeling good about yourself?

_____

_____

_____

_____

_____

_____

Now that you have thought about your inner critic and gremlin, have some fun giving this part of you a name: _____.

How did it feel to reflect on some of the things your inner critic and gremlin says to you? Think about how regularly these thoughts go through your head. Again, as tempting as it is to give your Gertrude the boot, it can be more helpful to keep them near you so you can keep a close eye on them.

Identifying Thoughts That Make You Feel Good

Once you have identified these negative messages, spend some time thinking about the positive messages—the ones that motivate you and keep you moving toward your own happiness in life.

Note: Identifying these thoughts that make you feel good is not just about "being positive" or ignoring the rest of your feelings that do not have to do with happiness.

It is important to be intentional about these thoughts that help and motivate you, because once you can identify them you can begin to internalize them. And the more you can do this, the more you crowd out the inner critic and gremlin voices. Here are some examples of thoughts that might make you feel good:

- You can do this.

- You deserve to be happy.

- It's important to believe in yourself.

- It's OK to try something to see whether you like it.

- You are smart enough to do this.

- If you do not succeed, you learn something about what you like and do not like.

- It's most important what you think about yourself.

- It's natural to compare yourself to others, but it can distract you from what you really want to do in life.

- You can get support to do this if you want.

- It's OK to take chances.

Can you see why these thoughts are more encouraging to you as an LGBTQ person than your inner critic's messages? Was there a thought or thoughts that really resonated with you? Regularly using these affirmations can really boost your resilience. Complete the next resilience practice to identify how these affirmations can keep you encouraged and moving in a direction of greater resilience and thriving.

RESILIENCE PRACTICE: Personal Feel-Good Mantras That Inspire You

After reading the preceding list of suggestions, what other encouragements can you think of that would motivate you to try new things, believe in yourself more, and feel more confident? You can think of this list as go-to personal mantras that keep you headed in a direction of feeling good about who you are and what you can do in the world. Think to yourself, "If I had a personal coach, what would that person say to me that would really make me feel good about myself and my capabilities?" Write your responses here:

_____

_____

_____

_____

_____

_____

Now read through these personal feel-good mantras. How does it feel to read these words of encouragement and affirmation? Write some of these mantras on index cards, or on the worksheet version of this exercise that's available at http://www.newharbinger.com/39461, and post them in places in your home, work, or school where you can see them regularly.

Read Sonali Sadequee's story of how her resilience is related to her inherent value and self-worth as an LGBTQ person.

How I remember my self-worth [and] value and protect my dignity as a queer person is an ongoing learning and fine-tuning process. I make sure I connect with my queer/trans friends on a regular basis and that I have a strong queer/trans community that I am a part of. I like to make sure that I value and uplift others, queer or not, and subconsciously hope and expect that others will do the same for me. A mind game I have come to embody to help me value myself is that I choose to believe that I am already valued and appreciated by default when I meet people—I like to operate by this "benefit of the doubt" attitude. Sometimes when I fear that my value is being minimized or dismissed, I am training myself to remember faster to speak up and communicate how I prefer to be treated instead—this is very challenging for me. I think the most powerful thing that has helped me remember my self-worth is my own pride in myself as a queer person, a spiritual person, a Muslim vegan yogi, a brown Bengali immigrant woman, etc. The more proud I am of my various identities, the easier it is to automatically value my worth, I have found. The more proud I have grown over the years of my queerness, the bolder I am in valuing the queer goddess that resides within me, across relationships and spaces.

—Sonali Sadequee, South Asian, queer,
cisgender woman

Assertiveness Training

Identifying the messages that are truly motivating and encouraging for you is a key building block in developing your self-confidence. That self-confidence is important for all people, and becomes critically important for queer and trans resilience. As mentioned earlier, queer and trans people are at more risk than the average population for various mental health challenges because of the often-frequent microaggressions and macroaggressions that LGBTQ people experience in society.

Research shows that over their life span, queer and trans people are the target of bullying in related to their gender identity and sexual orientation (Kosciw, Greytak, Giga, Villenas, & Danischewski, 2017). This bullying can range from covert and mild to overt and aggressive. Other research suggests that developing confidence and assertiveness skills for queer and trans people can be a protective factor for this type of harassment (Russell, Ryan, Toomey, Diaz, & Sanchez, 2011). I want to be clear: I'm not saying that people who are bullied for being LGBTQ are not confident or somehow deserve what they are experiencing. However, it's important to understand that learning to stand up for yourself and knowing what treatment you might expect from others can be a significant factor in building strong resilience.

This type of confidence development is often called assertiveness. There are numerous books, training programs, and online resources that can help you be more assertive. Each of these approaches to developing assertiveness makes a point of defining what assertiveness *is* and is *not*.

Assertiveness is:

- A skill that can be learned

- Helpful when communicating with others

- Needed when interacting with family members, friends, work and school peers, and in other interpersonal interactions, like in public spaces

- Useful to help you remember your value

- Helpful to keep you calm in stressful situations

Assertiveness is not:

- The same thing as being aggressive

- Ignoring other people's thoughts and feelings

- Being rigid with your expectations

- A onetime event

- Driven by fear

Keeping this in mind, let's read through some case scenarios to see how assertiveness can help you not only increase your self-esteem but also demonstrate that self-esteem when interacting with others.

Addressing use of wrong pronouns. A Latino trans man, Julio, is at a work meeting. One of his coworkers consistently uses the wrong pronouns to refer to Julio. Julio asks the coworker to speak with him after the meeting. Calmly, Julio shares with his coworker what his correct pronouns are and his expectation that his coworker will use them.

Asking for a safe LGBTQ space. A White gay man, Derek, has been at his college for three years. Over that time, he has made several friends in the LGBTQ community. However, there is no student group that is dedicated to queer and trans issues. Derek asks to meet with a student affairs administrator. He explains why the LGBTQ group is needed, as well as some of his own experiences as a gay college student.

Experiencing mistreatment. An African American trans woman, Leila, is a computer engineer working on a university campus. Leila is walking across campus for a meeting with another department when the university police stop her and tell her that only students can be on campus. Leila shows her university identification to the university police and asks, "What specific factors led you to think I did not belong on campus as a university personnel or student?" Afterward, she reports the incident to the chief of the university police.

Expecting to be treated well on a date. Dawn is a Native American, two-spirit person. They go on a date with Kevin, whom they met at the movies a week ago. When they meet their date at dinner, they have a good connection with Kevin. After dinner, Kevin asks Dawn to go to his place and have sex. Dawn shares they do not have sex with people they date until they get to know them better because their safety is important to them.

These case scenarios are a sampling of different situations where assertiveness can be not only helpful but also important to safety and feeling a sense of belonging and support in your community. As you read each scenario, did you have questions or think you might do things a little differently? If so, that is OK. Complete the next resilience practice to explore self-assertiveness further.

RESILIENCE PRACTICE: Developing a Personal Definition of Assertiveness

The goal of this resilience practice is to help you define what assertiveness means to you in a variety of settings. Answer the following questions based on different settings in which you might interact with people as a queer or trans person.

What would your assertiveness look like with your family members?

_____

_____

_____

_____

What would your assertiveness look like with your friends?

_____

_____

_____

_____

What would your assertiveness look like in your intimate relationships?

_____

_____

_____

_____

What would your assertiveness look like at work or school?

_____

_____

_____

_____

What would your assertiveness look like in public spaces?

_____

_____

_____

_____

As you answered each question, you might have noticed some repeating themes in terms of your assertiveness—ways in which standing up for yourself is really important. You also might have noticed that there are strengths and growing edges—the skills that you want to develop further—in your assertiveness as an LGBTQ person. The strengths are important to know about, as you can draw on them in challenging situations. The growing edges are also signifi-cant, as they are areas you can continue to think about and develop further so you feel more confident and prepared.

Taking Risks and Expanding Your Comfort Zone

In many ways, the act of growing your self-esteem entails taking risks and expanding your comfort zone. However, it can be helpful to more closely examine how taking calculated risks can enlarge your positive feelings about yourself and grow your self-confidence. Take a look at the figure on the following page for a visual portrayal of your comfort zone and how important it is to your self-esteem.

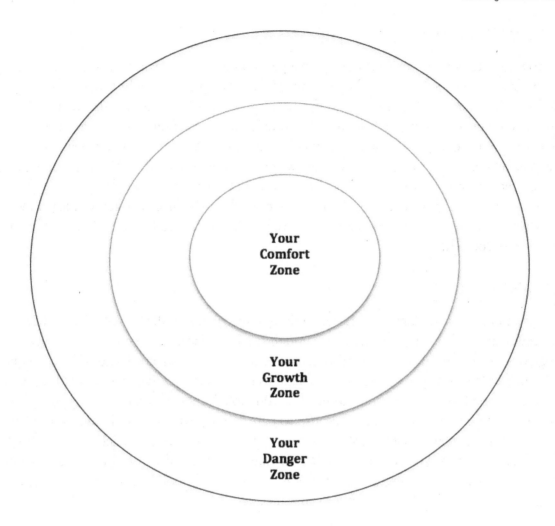

In the figure, each of the three concentric circles plays an important role in your resilience as an LGBTQ person. Let's talk more about these three zones.

COMFORT ZONE

This comfort zone is your home base. You feel safe here, and you like to hang out here. It is a good place to be when you feel tired, scared, angry, or even happy. A comfort zone is good to have, because you know really well what you like and do not like. However, a comfort zone can be stifling sometimes, as no new growth happens inside it. When no new growth happens, then your comfort zone can start to feel stale, rigid, and possibly reflective of an "old" you that has stopped growing. Examples might be hanging out with the same group of friends who do not challenge you to learn more about who you are and what you like. Your comfort zone is a good place to rest and regroup after spending time in the growth zone, so this home base is important for reflection and reassessment of your growth as well.

GROWTH ZONE

Your growth zone is where the magic happens! This is where you take some calculated risks to learn more about your world and yourself. For example, you might learn a new hobby, ask for a raise, start to date, move to a different location, or become more assertive and confident. There are endless ways to interact with your growth zone from your comfort zone. You know you are in your growth zone when you feel slightly scared, but not overwhelmed, about new possibilities and learnings. You also know you are in your growth zone when you take a risk and accomplish something and feel excited about future growth. The growth zone is where the magic happens because when you take a risk in the growth zone, you learn more about who you are and what you like and do not like, which thereby expands your comfort zone. Pretty cool, eh?

DANGER ZONE

Expanding your comfort zone through taking some risks is really cool. However, beyond the growth zone is the danger zone, which entails too much risk, to the point that it becomes dangerous to you. Just like the comfort and growth zones, each person's danger zone is unique to them. Sometimes things we can't control land us in the danger zone, like the sudden death of someone you love, or a relationship breakup. But you'll know you are in the danger zone when there is no growth happening because you are too overwhelmed and have no capacity to learn anything new about yourself. You may decide to move to a new city for a new job (growth zone), but may reach that city without asking friends and family for any personal or professional connections there (danger zone). Rather than expanding your comfort zone, you risk getting hurt and not looking out for yourself.

Life begins at the edge of your comfort zone.

—Neal Donald Walsh, White, cisgender man, author

Using Your Understanding of the Three Zones

Understanding how these three zones—comfort zone, growth zone, and danger zone—apply to you as an LGBTQ person can really enhance your resilience in many situations. When you learn to recognize which zone you are in at any given time, you've gained a great assessment tool. First, you can simply ask yourself: "Which zone am I in right now?" Then ask yourself, "Will being in this zone strengthen or weaken my resilience?" For example, you may realize you are in a danger zone where you are physically or emotionally unsafe (like feeling depressed). Strengthening your resilience in this situation means retreating to your growth or comfort zone (such as connecting with other people). Or you may ask yourself the question and realize you are playing it too safe (like staying in a school or job that is not LGBTQ-affirming), and that getting out of your comfort zone and into your growth zone (such as looking for a new LGBTQ-affirming school or job) will increase your resilience.

Sometimes, when it is difficult to answer these two questions, it's helpful to move back into your comfort or growth zones to stabilize yourself. Complete the following resilience practice to apply these three zones to your own life as an LGBTQ person.

RESILIENCE PRACTICE: Exploring Your Comfort, Growth, and Danger Zones

Think about your own comfort, growth, and danger zones. Which one do you tend to live in most? Are you someone who rarely takes risks, thereby risking little growth? Do you tend to live too much in your danger zone? Do you live most of the time in your growth zone, allowing little time in your comfort zone to recoup, rest, and make meaning of your growth? Across these zones, how does being LGBTQ affect your risk-taking?

How does being LGBTQ affect your comfort zone?

_____

_____

_____

_____

How does being LGBTQ affect your growth zone?

_____

_____

_____

_____

How does being LGBTQ affect your danger zone?

_____

_____

_____

_____

As you reflect on these three zones, you should feel more informed about how being a queer or trans person in this society affects you. Mostly, it is important to understand that LGBTQ stigma often threatens your resilience because you stop learning more about who you are and what you like. Identifying which zone you are in with any action or situation gives you a good indicator of whether it will support your resilience or weaken it. In terms of LGBTQ stigma, you can use this assessment to determine where you need to be in terms of risk-taking and keeping yourself safe. With regard to resilience, use the zone check to figure out where you want to take a risk and grow next.

I know that, as a bisexual, sometimes people who are gay or lesbian look down upon the bisexual community as well and assume that people who are bisexual just don't know what they want.

—Crystal Bowersox, White, cisgender,
lesbian woman and singer

Resilience Wrap-Up

Realizing your self-worth as a queer and trans person is a critical aspect of resilience, because when you increase your self-esteem, you increase your expectation that you will be treated with respect and dignity. Strengthening your self-esteem takes some work, but it's worth it. When you feel more positive about yourself, you can send a message to others that you will not tolerate mistreatment. Remember the following points:

- Self-worth and self-esteem are similar—they both refer to how you feel about yourself and what you believe you are capable of doing.

- It is important to nurture your general self-esteem, as well as your self-worth as an LGBTQ person.

- Naming your inner critic can help you notice when you are being hard on yourself—and challenge that gremlin voice.

- Intentionally identifying thoughts that motivate you to live a happy life is a part of resilience.

- Being assertive means being better able to advocate for yourself as an LGBTQ person and knowing what treatment to expect.

- You expand your comfort zone by taking calculated risks in your growth zone, and avoiding your danger zone where no growth can happen.

In Chapter 5, you'll move from the discussion of knowing your self-worth as an LGBTQ person to the resilience strategy of knowing how to stand up for yourself.

Standing Up for Yourself

In Chapter 4 you learned a good deal about self-esteem and valuing yourself as key parts of your resilience as an LGBTQ person. The more you feel good about yourself, the easier it is to know what treatment you should expect from others and when you should stand up for yourself and challenge injustice. This chapter continues this discussion, exploring how standing up for yourself, even in tough circumstances, can enhance your resilience. In the previous chapter you explored your inherent worth and dignity as a person; in this chapter you explore how to stand up for yourself as an LGBTQ person. In many ways, standing up for yourself is about developing healthy communication skills and knowing how to take actions that can help you advocate for yourself in a variety of settings.

Communication, Communication, Communication

In real estate, you will often hear agents talk about "location, location, location" to emphasize that when it comes to assessing a home's market value and determining an asking price, one factor is paramount: people are more drawn to a *place* they want to live—the street and surrounding neighborhood—than to the house itself. When it comes to standing up for yourself, the one paramount factor is communication, and that too is worth repeating! We'll have much more to say about that shortly.

You typically will stand up for yourself when *you know that you have value*, when *you know you are right*, and when *you know you have backup and support*.

Because it bears repeating, these are the three elements necessary to standing up for yourself:

- You believe your perspective has value.

- ou believe your perspective is right.

- You have the support you need.

Growing More Positive Self-Talk

Given these three necessary elements, the communication you have with yourself is a crucial part of standing up for yourself. However, most people don't get a crash course on how to have healthy communication with others, much less with ourselves! So, you may struggle—at a basic level—with how you communicate with yourself (that inner critic/gremlin inside of each of us that I talked about in Chapter 4). That is the first place to start building the resilience you need to stand up for yourself.

If you think about it, you are the person you spend the most time with in any given twenty-four hours. So the relationship you have with yourself is important! The self-talk inside of your head about yourself as an LGBTQ person or about any of your other identities influences your overall resilience. In the next resilience practice you can get a feel for how well you communicate with yourself.

RESILIENCE PRACTICE: How Positive Is My Inner Self-Talk?

The goal of this resilience practice (which is available in worksheet form at http://www.newhar binger.com/39461) is to rate how positively you communicate with yourself. What does that inner voice "sound like" in your head? In the first part of this resilience practice, you'll explore what positive self-talk you already have, as well as areas for your future growth. Then you'll reflect on which people can be models of positive self-talk for you.

Intrapersonal

Consider how often you think you use the following actions to get through hard times as an LGBTQ person, then check the column for your response for each.

	Never	Rarely	Sometimes	Often
Reflect on how you feel				
Feel good about yourself				
Use positive self-talk				
Manage your emotions				
Remind yourself of your self-worth				
Remember your strengths				

Feel OK about making mistakes				
Feel hopeful about your life				
Learn from your past				
Adapt to change				
Plan ahead for the future				
Put your plans into action				
Reach out for support				
Communicate how you are feeling				

What do you notice about your use of positive self-talk? What are the places where you are really strong, or need to grow, on the list? Take four different color highlighters to distinguish the items you assigned the four different frequencies. How can you use your strengths in intrapersonal resilience to help grow the actions that you never or rarely take? For example, if you often manage your emotions but rarely communicate how you are feeling, then you could start working on using your emotional management to help you more readily share how you are feeling.

This activity is meant to spark awareness of internal self-talk that you can change. Next, you'll explore your interpersonal resilience when you are communicating with others.

Models of Self-Talk

List the family, friends, teachers, mentors, online communities, and other people in your life who model positive LGBTQ self-talk to you. It's OK to list people you may not know personally or those you see only in the media.

_____

_____

_____

_____

_____

What are the specific positive self-talk statements you hear these people making?

_____

_____

_____

_____

_____

_____

Did you find it relatively easy or more challenging to identify people who communicate positive self-talk? What specific things do they say about themselves and others? Part of growing your resilience in terms of your self-talk is paying attention to how others communicate positively about themselves. These people can be positive reinforcers and reminders to speak to yourself with kindness, love, and appreciation. And remember, when you have positive self-talk, you are more skilled at standing up for yourself as an LGBTQ person.

Making Your Self-Talk More Resilient

Your resilience in terms of being able to stand up for yourself is not just about remaining positive. Actually, more positive self-talk sometimes does not seem that positive at all. You can think of it like an inner coach. A coach is not going to tell you that you are awesome for no reason. A coach is not going to lie to you, or pretend that there are no areas in which you need to grow and change. A coach is going to *be real with you* and tell you the truth. Not truth as in something to be hard on yourself about, but truth that will encourage you to believe that you are worth having dreams, meeting goals, and—you guessed it—sticking up for yourself. And ultimately, that inner coach is going to stand up for you in all situations—in good times and bad times—and will push you to be the best self you can be.

I once had a lot of negative self-talk about how I dressed. I thought that just because I was genderqueer, I had to wear more masculine clothes or fit into a certain stereotypical image. The more I challenged this underlying belief, the more free and affirmed I felt in my gender identity. And the more I did this, the more I felt like I could stand up for nonbinary identity as a valid and important part of who I am, even if people make lots of incorrect assumptions about my gender.

How do you shift your internal self-talk and develop the best inner coach ever? There are actually some simple steps, though they can seem tough to implement at times. The key is to practice, practice, practice.

Reframing Negative Thoughts

The first step in challenging our negative thoughts is to master the skill of *reframing*. Again, the point is not to just change a thought, but to recognize that there are some options for other thoughts as well. Why do thoughts matter, and is it really that simple? Well, in some ways, yep, it is. Your brain is pretty predictable. All of us have a lot of mental chatter inside of our heads (and most of it negative). Research has suggested that thoughts drive your feelings, so you can see why in a workbook about increasing your resilience as an LGBTQ person you will need to reflect on your innermost thoughts. These thoughts can drive your beliefs about standing up for yourself.

As a human, you may make some attribution errors about your inner thoughts. Put more simply, you blame your thoughts and feelings on other things. Those other things may be events in your life or things and people you can't control. You might believe that *events* or *people* cause your *feelings*.

Maybe you went to a *family event* and *everyone there made you feel unworthy*. Or, you are *stressed* because you were late to work or school because *the person in front of you* was driving slowly. I could go on and on. The thing is, I am not saying the family event was a great time and you should have just gotten through it the best you could, and I am not saying the person driving in front of you was driving fast enough. I am saying that the research I referenced earlier about thoughts driving your feelings proposes another step in the process of how you *feel* that does not include events or people. That step is your *thoughts*. Check this out:

> *Events* happen and *people* do things, and you have *thoughts* about these events and people and their actions, which drive your *feelings*.

Let's review that again. Something happens—an event occurs or a person in your life does something. You go to a family event, and the people there make anti-LGBTQ and racist remarks. You have some thoughts about this event and these people, like "This event is something I *have* to go to" or "These people *hate* me." Then your thoughts drive your feelings, which you are left with after being at the event and interacting with the people, such as feeling rejected or unworthy.

This new equation—that events and people's actions happen and your *thoughts* about them drive your feelings—is the best news in the world for your resilience as an LGBTQ person. Your inner coach can name the truth of what is going on with LGBTQ-negative environments and people and remind you that your thoughts can move you up the empowerment ladder (such as "I know going to this event may make me feel I am unworthy, but actually it is *their* LGBTQ-negative beliefs that they are expressing that are the problem, and I will remember that I think my gender identity and sexual orientation have value") or even help you make better decisions (such as "I will attend the family event for only an hour, because I want to feel good about myself when I leave").

Complete the next resilience practice to test a scenario in your own life with this thoughts-cause-feelings equation.

RESILIENCE PRACTICE: Notice How Your Thoughts Cause Your Feelings

The aim of this resilience practice is for you to explore how to stay grounded in thoughts related to your positive value as an LGBTQ person in a current situation in your life. Consider the following question: What is an example of an event that tends to be heterosexist or a person who tends to be a heterosexist? Write your responses to interactions at this event or with this person.

The event or person is:

_____

_____

What are your typical thoughts about this event or person?

_____

_____

_____

_____

What are your typical feelings as a result of these thoughts?

_____

_____

_____

_____

Did you notice how it is the thoughts you have, and not the events or people, who cause how you feel? What a relief! To be able to know that, in a world that is not always LGBTQ-affirming, you can identify negative thoughts that do not enhance or strengthen your resilience. This is a major key to resilience. And that's part of how you learn you are worth standing up for, more and more.

Now, let's get to the reframing part. Reframing your thoughts helps you be more resilient to hard times and situations, and it is important to remember that there may be a process of "moving up a ladder" of emotions in order to nurture your empowerment as an LGBTQ person. Consider the following example:

Event: You are walking down the street, and someone calls out an anti-LGBTQ epithet.

Thought: "What did I do wrong?"

Feeling: Depressed, despondent, sad.

Reframing means focusing on the thoughts as the site of change and action. Consider this reframing of the thought:

Event: You are walking down the street, and someone calls out an anti-LGBTQ epithet.

Thought: "What did I do wrong?" You catch yourself, and you shift your thought to, "That was a horrible thing this person did, and I did not deserve that treatment."

Feeling: Shift to determined, confident, grounded.

See how that happened? It is natural that you may have some initial self-defeating thoughts. However, the sooner you can catch yourself in the act of having those thoughts, the sooner you can shift your feelings back to those of self-worth, self-validation, and self-love as an LGBTQ person.

You can also dig deeper into the sequence, and notice that the following happens:

Event: You are walking down the street, and someone calls out an anti-LGBTQ epithet.

Thought: "What did I do wrong?"

Feeling: Depressed, despondent—on the sad end of the emotional spectrum.

Thought: You ask yourself, "What thought can I have that can shift my emotions to be more empowered?" You shift your thought to, "That was a horrible thing this person did, and I did not deserve that treatment."

Feeling: Your feelings shift to: determined, confident, grounded.

Use this resilience practice to apply reframing to another current situation in your life as an LGBTQ person and how you can stand up for yourself.

_____

Now you have the knowledge of how powerful your thoughts are in directing your feelings when it comes to being queer and trans. So if there are anti-LGBTQ messages coming at you from society in so many different areas, it is important to start training your mind to not only notice those thoughts, but also to challenge them. In the next resilience practice, you'll explore how to develop an LGBTQ-affirming inner voice.

_____

RESILIENCE PRACTICE: Using Reframing to Develop Your Inner Coach

The aim of this resilience practice (which is available in worksheet form at http://www.newhar binger.com/39461) is for you to practice strengthening that voice of your inner coach, who can help you reframe and challenge negative events and people that could decrease your resilience. Select another example of an event or a person's actions that presents an anti-LGBTQ message. Write your responses related to interactions at this event or with this person.

The event or person is: _____

_____

What are your typical thoughts about this event or person?

_____

_____

_____

_____

What are your typical feelings as a result of these thoughts?

_____

_____

_____

_____

What thoughts can you use to reframe this situation or interaction with this person and shift your feelings?

_____

_____

_____

_____

Digging deeper, what feelings would you like to have in this situation or in interactions with this person? What thoughts could shift you to these feelings?

_____

_____

_____

_____

_____

_____

In completing this exercise, did you see how powerful it is to shift a negative thought and reframe it so you are more grounded and feeling good about yourself? Did you understand how you can work backward from feelings you know you should have as an LGBTQ person, like feeling empowered, valued, and confident? Did you notice you want to stand up for yourself more in this situation? Was it easier to see why you should stand up for yourself as an LGBTQ person? It takes some practice, but the more you do this, the more resilient you will feel when facing LGBTQ-negative situations and people.

What Is Healthy Communication with Others?

You can probably already see that the ways you communicate with yourself can influence other interactions, including how you communicate in standing up for yourself with others. Healthy communication means, in essence, interactions with others in which you stay true to yourself, set boundaries, and build your connections with them. The stronger your communication skills with others, the more resilience you'll have to move through difficult times; because you value yourself, you trust that you can communicate your thoughts, feelings, and needs to others.

The core of healthy communication in relationships—whether with your partners, at work, at school, or with family and others—is being able to *listen to others* and to *express your thoughts and needs*. It means knowing the essentials of effective listening and talking.

Let's start with listening. Here are some general tips to show others that you are listening to them:

- Be present and pay attention—no multitasking, such as texting, while you are listening.

- Paraphrase what the talker is saying to show that you "heard" them.

- Demonstrate that you are open to listening to them.

- Show empathy by "stepping into their shoes" to understand what they are experiencing.

- If you are confused, ask questions, but don't interrupt.

- Practice!

One of the most sincere forms of respect is actually listening to what another has to say.

—Bryant H. McGill, White, cisgender, author

Just as there are listening skills, so too there are talking skills. The communication in your relationships should have a healthy balance between listening and talking. In Chapter 7, you will more deeply explore healthy communication with regard to your relational identity (for example, monogamous, polyamorous, aromantic). For now, here are some skills that will help you better express what you are feeling:

- Use "I" statements.

- Stay calm.

- Express feelings.

- Focus on solutions.

- Practice!

Communication with others can be more healthy when you already have a solid belief system that you are worth standing up for—whether it is your perspective, thoughts, feelings, ideas, or other things you would like to communicate with others. Standing up for yourself doesn't always include making the person you are communicating with believe your perspective is right. It just means that you value yourself enough to be your real self. Of course, this can get complicated in some situations—like if you feel unsafe in a relationship or haven't disclosed some parts of yourself to another. Standing up for yourself with others is also about making decisions about what is right and not right for you to share about your thoughts, feelings, ideas, and so on with others when interacting with them.

It is obviously difficult to practice listening and talking skills in a workbook—as you read by yourself, there is no chance for live interaction! However, the next resilience practice will help you think about your communication skills as both listener and speaker.

RESILIENCE PRACTICE: How Well Do You Communicate?

The goal of this resilience practice is for you to explore your communication. To the left of each statement, note whether you think you do this activity VW (very well), SW (somewhat well), or NW (not well).

Listening Skills

_____ Being present and paying attention to the listener.

_____ Paraphrasing what the talker is saying (when it's your turn!) to show that you've heard them.

_____ Demonstrating that you are open to hearing the person speaking.

_____ Showing empathy by "stepping into their shoes" to understand what they are experiencing.

_____ Asking questions if you are confused, but avoiding interrupting.

Speaking Skills

_____   Using "I" statements.

_____   Staying calm.

_____   Expressing your feelings.

_____   Focusing on solutions.

What did you notice about your listening and speaking strengths and growing edges? Were you surprised by your ratings? What growing edges could you work on developing in order to strengthen your resilience as an LGBTQ person, and what listening or speaking strengths can you rely on in furthering your resilience? Write about your strengths and growing edges in terms of your listening and speaking skills:

_____

_____

_____

_____

_____

_____

Now that you have reflected on both your strengths and your growing edges with healthy communication, you should have a good idea of a few areas you can work on to develop your resilience in this area.

There are lessons in everything—the bad, the good. Our job is to listen, and to continue to learn, so that maybe we get better at life.

—Laverne Cox, Black trans actress and activist

Decision-Making and Standing Up for Yourself

Up to this point in the chapter, you have learned how important communication is—intrapersonally, in terms of your inner coach, and interpersonally, in terms of how you speak and listen to others. These skills help you develop your resilience and feel grounded when you are interacting with yourself and with the world. Healthy communication skills also strengthen your relationships, as you have a solid foundation on which to make decisions as an LGBTQ person. This decision-making skill is a crucial foundation, as LGBTQ people face challenges and threats to their identities in a multitude of settings and relationships. Strong decision-making skills help you move through such adversity and determine the best choices for your overall well-being.

Some of these choices can be heartbreaking: as an LGBTQ person, you must prepare yourself to potentially experience discrimination in employment, schools, housing, government, and public settings, as well as your family, social circles, and religious and spiritual institutions. When you face these challenges, you are forced to make decisions—often in the moment, often when you are in shock, and often when you feel unprepared to do so. People make decisions all the time, but you know how challenging these potentially life-changing decisions can be, and how indecision and uncertainty can shift you away from your center. That's why working to develop your decision-making skills can help you stand up for yourself and what you know is right in terms of your own life and how you should be treated.

There is a myth about decision-making: that you just *decide*—and that doing so entails just one step. In actuality, there are multiple steps to making a decision. Here is a decision-making model I like to use when I face tough decisions:

- Identify the decision you need to make.

- Research information that can help you make this decision.

- Assess the possible alternatives.

- Name the pros and cons of these alternatives and the decision at hand.

- Act on the alternative with the most pros and the fewest cons.

- Step back and look at the alternative you selected, assessing whether it was the right one for you.

The next resilience practice helps you apply these decision-making steps to a situation in your current life.

RESILIENCE PRACTICE: Applying Decision-Making Skills to Your Life

The goal of this resilience practice (which is available in worksheet form at http://www.newhar binger.com/39461) is for you to apply the decision-making skills just listed to some practical need in your life. Think about the last time you faced a hard decision as an LGBTQ person. With that example in mind, respond to the following questions related to each decision-making step:

What was the decision you needed to make?

_____

_____

_____

_____

What information did you research that helped you make this decision?

_____

_____

_____

_____

How did you assess the possible alternatives to this decision?

_____

_____

_____

_____

What were the pros and cons of these alternatives?

_____

_____

_____

_____

Did you act on the decision with the most pros and the fewest cons?

_____

_____

_____

_____

Did you step back and look at the alternative you selected, assessing whether it was the right one for you?

_____

_____

_____

_____

How did you feel thinking about this decision you made? Did you see different possibilities? Were there steps you did not take, but would take if you had another opportunity to decide? Can you see how a decision can be composed of multiple steps? Practice using these steps to help slow down in situations where you feel pressured to make a decision as an LGBTQ person, or you experience threats to your resilience. This can offer you time to get support and remind yourself that as an LGBTQ person you are a valuable and important part of society and are deserving of a thoughtful decision-making process.

If I didn't define myself for myself, I would be crunched into other people's fantasies for me and eaten alive.

—Audre Lorde, Black lesbian poet, writer,
and activist

Resilience Wrap-Up

In this chapter, you learned the different components of standing up for yourself as a part of your resilience, including:

- Knowing that communication, communication, communication is key!

- Understanding that communication with your own self is the foundation of standing up for yourself. If you believe you are worthy, you can stand up for yourself more easily.

- Having models of people with strong inner coaches who help reframe negative self-talk.

- Learning that events and people do not cause your feelings; rather, your thoughts cause your feelings.

- Developing strong listening and speaking skills when communicating with others.

- Knowing that decision-making skills entail not just one step, but several.

After reading this chapter, you should have a stronger sense of how to stand up for yourself and express yourself. In Chapter 6, you will spend time reflecting on your relationship with your own body and how to be more resilient through developing body positivity as an LGBTQ person.

Affirming and Enjoying Your Body

In the last few chapters, you explored how your resilience increases as you come to know your self-worth as an LGBTQ person, and you strengthened your communication skills. This chapter will guide you to learn how you feel about your body and how these feelings can influence various aspects of your life. From the messages you have picked up about your body to the feelings you *want* to have about your body, you will develop resilience practices to develop body-positive skills. I also talk about sex positivity, and how you may decide whether and when to share your body with others. In doing so, you will think about not only what you may or may not like, but also what you want to learn more about, and what isn't OK for your body when you share it with others. You will also have an opportunity to learn more about the diverse relational structures of LGBTQ people.

What Being Body Positive Actually Means

So what is body positivity? Some possible words may immediately come to mind. Body positivity consists of affirming thoughts, feelings, and actions about your body. The more body positive you are, the greater your resilience, because you learn to actively value your body and who you decide to share your body with.

Body positivity is especially important for LGBTQ people, as we often internalize negative messages about our community, and these same negative attitudes can then play out in how we think and feel about our body. Here is an example from my life. My ancestors are from northern India and Scotland, and it is in my DNA to have a larger belly. As I was learning more and more about my identity as a queer teenager, I also was experiencing all of these transformations in my body. As I learned that it wasn't safe for me to disclose my queer identity with most people, I also was learning negative attitudes about my body from the world at large. Any time I consumed media, I saw images in the magazines and on television that prized this image of a straight, White, super-feminine, cisgender, thin woman. I didn't have someone whispering in my ear or telling me directly that my body was amazing and important, and that

I should value my body. So it took me years to accept, appreciate, and (now) love my body for all that it can do, be, and look like on any given day. Sound familiar?

Before we go further, it is important to understand that body positivity does not mean that you love your body all of the time, or that you have to be engaging in positive thoughts, feelings, and actions about your body all of the time. Learning to be body positive is a process, not a final fixed outcome. The goal is to learn to appreciate your body, be kind to your body, and be able to identify when you are receiving negative messages about your body from others or yourself. That is what body positivity really means. To get you started, here are some examples of body-positive messages:

- My body is healthy and strong.

- I value my body.

- I love my body.

- I want to treat my body with the highest regard.

- I expect others to treat my body with the highest regard.

- There are lots of different body types, and mine is awesome.

- I own my own body and am in charge of what happens to it.

- A scratch or a scar is proof that I have lived my life and that my body can heal.

- I work out so I can sleep better, take care of myself, and feel good.

- I eat foods that nourish me and that I love.

- I love the body that I am in right now.

- My body changes with each day, but it is always mine to take care of and value.

These are just a few examples of body-positive statements! And it's OK if many of them seemed really familiar to you because you believe them—or if you weren't sure whether you could believe them or trust that you could feel these ways about your body. Either way is completely fine, because taking some time to reflect on your relationship with your body is a big part of your resilience. Complete the next resilience practice to explore your relationship with your own body, which is the first step in body positivity: to be aware of your thoughts, feelings, and actions toward your body.

RESILIENCE PRACTICE: How Do You Typically Feel about Your Body?

In this resilience practice, you'll explore how body positive you are as a queer or trans person. Remember, body positivity isn't an outcome, or even a thing you can make happen overnight. It's a process. So as you work through the following questions, you'll explore how you generally think, feel, and act in relation to your body. Your answers will create a mini-compass for how to develop more body positivity as an LGBTQ person.

What typical thoughts and feelings do you have about your body?

_____

_____

_____

_____

_____

How do these typical thoughts and feelings influence how you treat your body?

_____

_____

_____

_____

_____

Who and what were (or are) the major influences on how you treat your body?

_____

_____

_____

_____

_____

Overall, when it comes to those thoughts, feelings, and actions, do you think you are more body positive or body negative?

_____

_____

_____

_____

_____

As you responded to these questions, how did you feel? Were you surprised by anything that you wrote about the influences on your body? Did you realize you are more body positive, body negative, or some of both? Does that change based on who you are around or messages you receive as an LGBTQ person? In the next section we'll take a closer look at what it means specifically to be body positive as an LGBTQ person.

LGBTQ Body Positivity

As mentioned earlier, being body positive can be challenging for queer and trans people, because we may already be dealing with negative social attitudes toward us, and on top of that there may not have been a ton of people in our lives teaching us how to be body positive. For these reasons, exploring what it means to be body positive as an LGBTQ person is especially significant.

You can pick up negative messages about your body not just in the outside world, but also within the LGBTQ community. There has been a good deal of research, for instance, examining body image within cisgender gay men's communities, specifically of how a certain body type is prized, which community members are expected to strive for to be considered attractive. Trans people face pervasive media messages about what being a man or woman should look like, and nonbinary and genderqueer people are also influenced by these body-negative messages.

In addition, as you learned in Chapter 2, you have more identities than just gender and sexual orientation. So you can pick up body-negative messages within cultural groups as well. Latinx, cisgender, and trans lesbian women may pick up sexualized messages about their bodies; Asian American–Pacific Islander LGBTQ people may face being called "exotic" and other descriptors. In the following resilience practice, you get to explore body positivity and resilience strategies to counter internalizing these messages.

RESILIENCE PRACTICE: Being Body Positive as an LGBTQ Person with Multiple Identities

This resilience practice guides you to explore how your body positivity, LGBTQ identity, and other identities all come together. Respond to the following prompts:

As an LGBTQ person, how do you feel about your body?

_____

_____

_____

_____

What specific messages have you received about your body—or bodies in general—from within LGBTQ communities?

_____

_____

_____

_____

_____

113

What specific messages have you received about your body—or bodies in general—from within a cultural group related to one or more of your other identities, such as race/ethnicity, disability, and social class?

_____

_____

_____

_____

_____

_____

Did it feel different to write about your exploration of messages related to your body within LGBTQ communities and other cultural groups versus those from the larger society? Did you hear some messages in various LGBTQ communities and cultural groups that were affirming, encouraging, and aimed toward body positivity? If so, how can those messages help you foster your resilience related to body positivity? This exploration sets you up to take a deeper dive into specific body-negative thoughts you may have about your body and how to shift them toward body-positive thoughts that increase your resilience.

Growing Your Body Positivity as an LGBTQ Person

In Chapters 3 and 5 you learned about shifting your thoughts in a more positive direction as a way to shift your feelings and increase your resilience. When you seek to grow your body positivity as an LGBTQ person, you can work with your thoughts in a similar manner. In this case the "events" are body-negative messages, such as the following list of examples. These are extremely body-negative messages; I list them so you can consider thoughts you may have had that are similar to or different from these:

- I am too fat.

- I should look like a "real" woman.

- Cisgender gay men like only other cisgender men.

- Lesbian women like only women with certain anatomy.

- I have to work out with weights to be considered attractive.

- I need to lose some weight.

- No one will think my body is attractive.

You get the idea. These are the kinds of thoughts that often run through our heads unconsciously. Let's see what it would be like to intentionally shift these thoughts to be more body positive:

- I appreciate my body and what it can do.

- There are some things I really enjoy about my body.

- I want to share my body with someone who will treat it with respect, dignity, and care.

- I am learning how to be more kind to my body.

- I get support when I get into a bad place with how I feel about my body.

See the difference in the two lists? The first list contains the messages you tend to pick up from society and internalize. The second list contains the messages that you should have been raised hearing or having someone teach you.

In the following resilience practice you'll explore how to increase your body positivity and resilience.

RESILIENCE PRACTICE: Building Body-Positive Resilience

In this resilience practice, you will identify how to shift body-negative messages you have internalized to intentionally building more body-positive messages as an LGBTQ person. You will list three body-negative thoughts and then identify a body-positive message you would like to begin using as a more affirming alternative.

List one body-negative thought you have as a queer or trans person.

_____

_____

What have been the major influences on this body-negative thought in terms of people, media, or something else?

_____

_____

What is a body-positive thought you would like to develop to replace this body-negative thought?

_____

_____

Who can support you in developing this more affirming body-positive thought?

_____

_____

Now identify a second body-negative thought and answer the same questions:

List one body-negative thought you have as a queer or trans person.

_____

_____

What have been the major influences on this body-negative thought in terms of people, media, or something else?

_____

_____

What is a body-positive thought you would like to develop to replace this body-negative thought?

_____

_____

Who can support you in developing this more affirming body-positive thought?

_____

_____

Identify a third body-negative thought and respond to the following prompts:

List one body-negative thought you have as a queer or trans person.

_____

_____

What have been the major influences on this body-negative thought in terms of people, media, or something else?

_____

_____

What is a body-positive thought you would like to develop to replace this body-negative thought?

_____

_____

Who can support you in developing this more affirming body-positive thought?

_____

_____

Was it hard to shift your body-negative thoughts to be more body positive? When you started to revise those thoughts, did you feel an emotional resistance or a feeling of hopelessness? Or was it relatively straightforward and easy for you to identify new, more affirming thoughts? Lastly, were your body-negative thoughts more related to your LGBTQ identity alone, several of your identities, or something else? These questions, again, are so important to your body positivity, which contributes to your overall resilience. This may seem like a simple activity, but consider what it would be like to really commit to building these new body-positive thoughts.

It takes some practice, for sure, but when you hear those body-negative thoughts in your head and catch them when they happen, be kind to yourself. Simply acknowledge the thoughts, then use some of your energy to say the new thought to yourself, even if you don't believe it now. As you practice this shift over time (perhaps using the worksheet version of this exercise that's available at http://www.newharbinger.com/39461), you will come to feel committed to treating your body well. After a day, week, month, or longer of shifting your thoughts, you can see how your resilience naturally develops over time.

Next, you will explore considerations in sharing your body with others.

Sex Positivity: Intimacy and Diverse Relational Structures

As you explore your relationship with your body and how to make decisions about whether to share your body with others or not, you may begin to consider dating, intimacy, and other forms of relationships. Each can be both exciting and stressful to think about and pursue. LGBTQ people can experience more stress than straight and cisgender people when it comes to these things, as so many feel pressure to hide who they are and who they have affection for and/or love, so resilience is important to develop in these areas.

To develop resilience in these areas, you can learn more about what relational structures are right for you. No matter the level or focus of your interest in sex or how you define intimate relationships for yourself, there are a variety of diverse relationship possibilities. Monogamy refers to relational structures of two partners who typically partner with only one another over a long time period. When it comes to monogamy, LGBTQ people may face a stereotype that they cannot be faithful in monogamy or don't have lasting monogamous relationships. However, many LGBTQ people, as far back as recorded history can tell us, have engaged in monogamy and have successful long-term relationships.

Polyamory refers to relational structures in which there may be more than two partners in a relationship. Within a polyamorous relationship, there may be two partners who are primary or "anchor" partners but have dating and/or sexual relationships with other people as well. In these primary partner relationships, there can also be freedom to have relationships outside of the anchor partnership that range from short term, like one sexual encounter, to long term, or somewhere in between. These are just a few examples of what polyamorous relationships can look like in real life. Polyamorous folks face myths as well—for example, that there is too much jealousy and that these relational structures don't last. Again, these are just myths. All relationships—whether monogamous or polyamorous, whether dating or engaging in a long-term relationship that may include cohabiting—require healthy communication. In the next resilience practice, you'll explore more about your identity related to diverse relational structures.

RESILIENCE PRACTICE: What Is Your Relational Identity?

In this resilience practice, you reflect on your own relational identity. Write your responses to the following prompts:

What relationship structures did you see growing up?

_____

_____

_____

_____

How would you describe your relational identity—monogamous, polyamorous, or something else?

_____

_____

_____

_____

What does it mean to you to have this relational identity as an LGBTQ person? Are there myths about your relational identity that you need to challenge?

_____

_____

_____

_____

_____

What aspects of your relational identity—such as developing healthy communication skills or how your relational identity is evolving—would you like to explore further?

_____

_____

_____

_____

_____

As you were doing this exercise, did you feel like you knew your responses right away or that you needed to think more about any of the questions in order to describe your relational identity? Relational identities are fluid, just like sexual orientation and gender identity in some ways. So keeping an open mind for learning about yourself and what is important to you emotionally, and possibly sexually, is the real key to being sex positive and increasing your resilience. Your resilience increases as an LGBTQ person when you have some time to explore and challenge any myths or negative attitudes about your relational identity that you may have realized. Then you can make healthier decisions about how to have intimate relationships—and whether you want to.

Doing personal work to affirm your body is a significant contributor to your resilience, and body positivity can help you make decisions about whether you would like to share your body with others. Sex positivity refers to the self-affirming decisions you make about sharing your body with others. For instance, you might be interested in intimate relationships, like dating and having sexual relationships. Or you may identify as asexual or aromantic, and sexual intimacy and relationships may be less of an interest for you.

Sex Positivity and Healthy Communication

As an overall note on this sex positivity section, depending on your age and your experiences with sex, you may want to get support in exploring sex positivity and healthy communication. It's important to make healthy decisions about whether to engage in intimate relationships, whether you are monogamous, polyamorous, or asexual, or have other sexual orientation identities. Across these relational and sexual orientation identities, communicating about a decision not to have sex is also an important skill. Although this workbook is not focused on sexual health, I touch on this topic because our sexual health does inform our resilience and overall well-being. Depending on your age and your experiences with sex, you may want to explore this topic further through other readings and discussions with supportive people in your life.

Communication and sexual health do go hand and hand, and for LGBTQ people sometimes it is already a huge endeavor to validate yourself and express yourself as an LGBTQ person. By the time you manage to do this, sexual health communication may be the last thing you talk about with supportive people, or it may be challenging to find people you can talk to about this.

So when we speak of sex positivity and communication we don't mean only the communication you have with others you decide to share your body with—or not—in intimate relationships. It is essential that you also get the LGBTQ-affirming information and support you need. I remember when I had no one to talk about sex with as a queer and nonbinary person, I had some amazing friends who were willing to practice communication with me. I was so worried at the time about how I would date; I had no idea what I would say or do—or was expected to say or do—as an LGBTQ person in developing intimate relationships.

With my friends, I was able to play out some scenarios and get important information about safer sex and started to think about what I might like when I decided to share my body with others. Then I felt more empowered. For instance, if you identify as asexual or aromantic, you may have been told "That isn't a real identity" or "You just haven't met the right person." Notice the similarity to what LGBTQ people hear as well! Feeling empowered in your identity can help you externalize these myths and validate your sex positivity and communication skills. Read Marla Stewart's take on her resilience and sex positivity as an LGBTQ person.

As a fierce lover and a Black, queer femme fighting for all marginalized folks, I find it very important to play as hard as I work. Because I'm dedicated to liberation of all kinds, but especially sexual liberation, giving and receiving pleasure is an undeniable act of resilience. Loving my body at every size that I've been and taking naked erotic selfies fill me with the light that I exude. I love being flirty, seducing strangers, and laughing with the people that I adore and love deeply; these are revolutionary acts because they involve a confident vulnerability that allows people to see me and recognize the love they have for themselves. Sex positivity is valuable, my sexual liberation is treasured, and my pleasure takes priority. This is how I stand in the world—bold, balanced, and brilliant.

—Marla Stewart, African American, queer,
cisgender, poly woman and activist

If you want to engage in sexual intimacy, it's important to imagine the scenarios that require you to make decisions and communicate what you want and don't want. Let's explore this further in the next resilience practice.

RESILIENCE PRACTICE: Communicating about Sharing—or Not Sharing—Your Body with Others

This resilience practice will guide you to reflect on what is important to you in terms of sex-positively communicating how you want to interact with others in an intimate manner.

When you think about communicating with another person about sharing your body (or not) with them, what thoughts and feelings come to mind?

_____

_____

_____

_____

Have you reflected on what you like and do not like with regard to intimate relationships when it comes to sharing your body (or not) with others?

_____

_____

_____

_____

What would help increase your resilience in terms of communicating to others about your body when you decide to share it (or not) with others?

_____

_____

_____

_____

In situations where you do not want to share your body with another person, what words would you want to use with this person? Think of this as an "elevator speech" and write it here.

_____

_____

_____

_____

As you completed this resilience practice, notice areas of communication in intimate relationships that you want to work on further, as well as areas that feel solid and strong to you. Overall, you want to use your strengths in communicating in a sex-positive way about what you like and don't like when sharing your body with others or not. Then you want to leverage those strengths in working on your growing edges when it comes to these decisions. Your resilience as an LGBTQ person grows when you do this.

Resilience Wrap-Up

In this chapter you've explored body positivity and sex positivity, two important aspects of enjoying your body, and learned these keys to resilience in this area:

- Developing body positivity is a process, not just an outcome goal.

- Identifying your body-negative thoughts and shifting them in a direction of affirming your body increases your resilience.

- Practicing body positivity messages is not just about loving your body and being positive all of the time; it's also about identifying ways to be more kind to yourself.

- Developing an affirming relationship with your body can help you make decisions about who you want to share your body with in intimate relationships, or whether you want to share your body at all.

- There are many diverse relational structures, as well as myths that LGBTQ people face concerning their relational identity.

- Monogamous and polyamorous relationships are most successful when the people involved emphasize healthy communication.

This chapter was all about the resilience you can develop when you pay attention to and learn about your body. In Chapter 7, you build on some of these ideas as you explore the resilience you can grow in building relationships and creating community for yourself as an LGBTQ person.

Building Relationships and Creating Community

When you know how to develop relationships and build a community that is supportive to you as a queer or trans person, you build your resilience and ability to move through tough times. In Chapter 5, you learned about healthy communication skills involving listening and speaking. We dive further into this topic in this chapter. Why is this important? Having healthy relationships helps support your resilience as a queer or trans person. You'll explore the skills you need to build strong relationships—like how to develop friendships, establish boundaries, and maintain the important relationships that encourage you.

In addition, you'll explore how you can create community as an LGBTQ person. Beyond reaching out for support and getting to know your community resources, it's important to build community for yourself. Building relationships and community is a very personal endeavor; it includes taking a closer look at your families of origin and possibly building families of choice that can help you be resilient and thrive.

Relationships and Well-Being

A large part of your everyday mental health comes from your relationships. These are a mix of those you may have had no choice about—your family, your school, your neighbors—and those you develop by choice, like your friends, your partners, and your work colleagues.

These relationships can either challenge or support your everyday mental health and overall well-being as an LGBTQ person. It's true: your mental health is as good as the quality of your relationships. That is where it gets complicated when it comes to your resilience as a queer or trans person. You may have experienced a good deal of oppression related to these or other identities in your various relationships, which clearly influences your overall mental health and well-being. Complete the following resilience practice to explore an important current relationship.

RESILIENCE PRACTICE: Exploring Your Resilience in an Important Relationship

In this resilience practice, think about a current relationship that means a lot to you as an LGBTQ person. This is a person you trust absolutely, who offers you steadfast encouragement. Write your answers to the following prompts.

Why is this particular person important to you as an LGBTQ person?

_____

_____

Is this person a friend, family member, work colleague, school peer, or someone else?

_____

List three ways that this supportive person has helped you be resilient as an LGBTQ person.

_____

_____

_____

What did you notice as you thought about this important relationship? Did you end up selecting a friend, family member, work colleague, school peer, or someone else to write about? Were there any themes in the three ways this person supports you? What could you learn about these themes for your other relationships?

On the other hand, it might have been difficult for you to identify even one person who encourages you as an LGBTQ person. Or you may have been able to think of only one or two ways in which this person supports you. If you currently have little direct support as an LGBTQ person, this chapter is particularly important for helping you begin developing relationships and building community that affirms you. If this resilience practice was pretty easy, that's OK too. You will have some opportunities to review how to maintain healthy relationships.

Whether this resilience practice was simple or challenging, it is important to think about your relationships. Queer and trans people often are just trying to get through the day as they come to understand their identities. You may have little chance to slow down and think about the *quality* of those relationships and how you develop them, much less the fact that you can choose to end unhealthy relationships. Next, you will learn more about the range of potential relationships and how to develop ones that are healthy for you as an LGBTQ person.

What Is a Relationship?

When you hear the word "relationship," like many people you may picture a dating relationship. However, relationships include a wide variety of connections, from friendships and intimate relationships to relationships with family, as well as with work and school peers or in other settings.

Within each of these categories you may feel varying depths of connection with someone. For instance, there are casual, more surface friendships, and those friendships where you feel you can share your deepest thoughts and challenges without judgment. Intimate relationships can range from dating and partnership to monogamy, polyamory, and romantic friendships, among other relational structures (discussed in Chapter 6). Other relationships also range in the level of depth of support you may experience as an LGBTQ person, such as a relationship with a religious/spiritual leader, your work supervisor, or a teacher/professor. In the next resilience practice you'll take an inventory of the wide range of your current relationships.

RESILIENCE PRACTICE: Take a Relationship Inventory

In this resilience practice (which is available in worksheet form at http://www.newharbinger .com/39461), inventory your current relationships to see the range of relationship types. For each type, place a check on the left and write the name(s) on the right. There are some spaces to add any types of current relationships not listed.

☐ Family relationships _____

☐ Extended family relationships _____

☐ Acquaintance relationships _____

☐ Friendship relationships _____

☐ School relationships _____

☐ Work relationships _____

☐ Sports relationships _____

☐ Religious/spiritual relationships _____

☐ Dating relationships _____

☐ Monogamous relationships _____

☐ Polyamorous relationships _____

☐ Romantic friendship relationships _____

☐ _____ relationships _____

☐ _____ relationships _____

☐ _____ relationships _____

☐ _____ relationships _____

☐ _____ relationships _____

In taking this inventory of your relationships, what did you notice? Did you have many or few of the relationship types that were listed? Did you write in additional types of relationships? Did you need additional space, because there were so many? Again note that some relationships have to do with things we can choose, like friendships and dating, while others we may not have choices about, such as family. Still others—at school and work, for example—may fall somewhere in between your having a complete choice whether to develop them or not. How did you feel overall about your inventory? Did you see areas you feel happy about and have worked hard to develop? Were there some gaps or types of relationships you would like to develop? Hold on to those thoughts as you explore how to develop relationships.

Developing Healthy Relationships

Because relationships are such a big part of your resilience, taking time to learn about how to develop healthy relationships is truly an investment in your overall mental health and well-being. Relationships are healthy when the person:

- Affirms your multiple identities as an LGBTQ person

- Supports your growth as a person

- Refrains from judgment

- Seeks to understand your experience

- Provides space to have disagreements and to reconnect

- Offers opportunities to trust one another more deeply

- Offers warmth and encouragement

- Enjoys shared similarities

- Strives to understand differences

- Provides a space of acceptance and positive regard

- Offers a point of view different from your own

- Celebrates accomplishments and triumphs

- Gives support during especially difficult times

- Provides accountability and support for self-care

You get the idea! Healthy relationships remind you of who you are and affirm you, but also challenge you to grow into an even better version of yourself.

Culturally Embedded Notions of Healthy Relationships

The conception of a healthy relationship can shift depending on the cultural worldview with which you were raised. In my culture, I was taught that family came first, before everything else. So as a queer person I did not reveal my sexual orientation and gender identity exploration to my family. I needed my own privacy and space to explore these parts of me with my chosen friendships. For myself, I realized over time that I appreciated the South Asian and Southern influences on my idea of a healthy relationship, because I value my family relationships greatly. At the same time, I also shifted my values in terms of what was healthy in my relationship with my family. So now I put my family first in some instances—when it enhances my overall well-being and mental health—and think carefully about doing this when that might mean neglecting what I need to be resilient and thrive as an LGBTQ person.

Sometimes the culture (or cultures) we grew up with is harder to identify, but as I noted in Chapter 2, a person's culture may encompass many identities. Complete the following resilience practice to explore how your image of a healthy relationship has been influenced by cultural influences growing up.

RESILIENCE PRACTICE: How Do Cultural Values Shape Your Ideas of Healthy Relationships?

This resilience practice will help you explore some possibly unexpected ways that your cultural upbringing has influenced your ideas of what should happen in good relationships. Consider the following questions and respond:

How would you describe your own culture?

_____

_____

_____

_____

_____

What messages did you receive about how you should engage in relationships based on your culture?

_____

_____

_____

_____

_____

Do you think you learned healthy ideas about relationships based on your culture growing up, or did you receive unhealthy ideas about relationships, or a mix of both?

_____

_____

_____

_____

_____

_____

How do these cultural messages influence how you develop relationships as an LGBTQ person?

_____

_____

_____

_____

_____

_____

Was it challenging to describe your culture, or was it relatively easy? Are there cultural messages about relationships that you want to retain, revise, or get rid of altogether? Remember, you get to decide which parts of your culture affirm you as an LGBTQ person, and sometimes this is complicated. For now, you are just assessing the culturally embedded messages about relationships that have influenced you, as well as how these might affect how you develop relationships today.

Developing Friendships

We took a closer look at intimate relationships in Chapter 6, but now let's dive into starting friendships. Some people call these relationships our "chosen family," depending on the depth of the friendship. Friendships entail all of the healthy qualities we listed in the beginning of the "Developing Healthy Relationships" section. Making friends, however, can seem a bit mysterious. Sometimes it just happens—you feel an instant connection with someone and you want to get to know them better. Other times, you meet people with whom you share interests such as hobbies or sports. Still other times, you may develop some of your closest relationships within the LGBTQ community, another group that shares your identity, or a shared experience, like school or work.

Although you can develop friendships in a variety of ways, most of us learn to rely on just a few approaches. In the next resilience practice, you'll explore the patterns in how you develop friendships.

RESILIENCE PRACTICE: Taking a Peek at Your Friend-Making Patterns

In this resilience practice, you reflect on the most common ways you tend to develop friendships. Think about how you formed your closest friendship and respond:

How did you first meet this friend? Were you the first to approach your friend, or vice versa?

_____

_____

_____

_____

_____

_____

How long did it take you to form a connection with this person?

_____

_____

_____

_____

_____

When did you realize this would be a close friendship?

_____

_____

_____

_____

_____

How do you think being extroverted, introverted, or somewhere in the middle played into developing this friendship? (You will learn more about introversion and extroversion in the next section.)

_____

_____

_____

_____

_____

When you think of other friendships you have developed in the recent past, what are the similarities and differences in how you made friends with this person?

_____

_____

_____

_____

_____

_____

What patterns did you notice in how you developed your friendship with the person you selected, as well as other friendships? Your exploration of how your personality might have played a role in developing this relationship can be good information for developing relationships in the future. Think about how these typical friendship-making patterns might influence how you develop friendships. This is good information, especially as it relates to the next section, in which you will reflect on your boundaries in friendships.

BOUNDARY SETTING

Boundary setting is a crucial step not only in making friends, but also in developing deeper and more connected relationships. What are boundaries? We touched on these briefly in Chapter 1. You can think of boundaries as delineating and protecting your own separate space from others. In your own space, you get to say what is OK and not OK in terms of how you are treated, such as how you are spoken to or interacted with in any relationship. Because LGBTQ people experience a good deal of discrimination, boundaries in the relationships you develop are especially important to express how you value yourself. When you express your boundaries to another in a friendship, it is an opportunity to notice how the other person reacts and whether your overall discussion of your boundaries helps bring you closer together.

How do you know your boundaries are being crossed in a relationship? Typically, you will feel uncomfortable. A part of you may want to ignore it or minimize a boundary intrusion, or you may feel a strong emotion like anger, sadness, or fear that lets you know something is not OK in this interaction with your friend.

Think of a friend you have known for a month and with whom you would like to develop a deeper connection. Now think about these situations with that person. Let's say you feel that a friend is asking questions that are too personal for you, or you feel the friend is somehow taking advantage of you. What do you think your reaction would be? Would you ignore your feelings? Would you ask to talk about how you feel? Would you share your emotions about the interaction with your friend? Most people follow a couple of different patterns in their responses to such boundary-crossing, just as they do in developing a friendship. Complete the next resilience practice to further explore how you express your boundaries.

RESILIENCE PRACTICE: Expressing Boundaries in Friendship to Deepen the Relationship

In this resilience practice, you will reflect on how you set boundaries through a personal example.

Think of a time you felt a friend had crossed your boundaries, and write about that experience.

_____

_____

_____

_____

How did you react to the boundary-crossing? Did you directly address it with your friend or not, and why did you choose to do so or not?

_____

_____

_____

_____

If you did directly address this boundary-crossing, what was the result? If you did not, what was that like for you afterward?

_____

_____

_____

_____

As you completed this resilience practice, could you feel the emotions you felt at the time of the boundary-crossing? Reflecting back on what you did or did not do, how do you feel? Would you do things differently if you had a chance to address this again? In the future, what might help you express your boundaries with your friends? How can what you learned about yourself in this resilience practice help you think about boundary setting in other relationships?

Maintaining Friendships

It may be weird to think about, but getting really good at boundary setting will help you not only maintain and deepen your current friendships, but also develop high-quality friendships that support you as an LGBTQ person in the future. Practice does make perfect! Make a habit of noticing when something feels OK, or not OK, to you in your friendships. Take a risk and communicate to your friend about it. Your healthiest friendships will deepen when you do so, because you have a chance to understand one another further through learning more about what is important to you both in your interactions. So having boundaries and setting them helps you increase your resilience. Boundaries are a two-way street—when you get good at setting your own boundaries, you start to look forward to learning more about your friends' boundaries as well. Just as it's important to develop friendships that can support you as an LGBTQ person, it's equally important to develop community as a queer or trans person. You'll learn about this next.

Building Community as an LGBTQ Person— One Step at a Time

In the LGBTQ world, people often throw around the word "community" quite a bit, but what is it, really? You can think of community as the networks of friendships, acquaintances, colleagues, peers, and others that share similar values and ways of looking at the world. Having community is more than just having access to resources and networks, although those aspects are important, as we discussed in the last chapter. Being a part of a supportive community is an important component of resilience, as the community can support you when things are rough—like when anti-trans legislation passes or when queer youth experience discrimination in schools. LGBTQ communities are not the only communities you may feel—or want to feel—you are a part of, but there are times it can be particularly important to be part of an LGBTQ-affirming community. In such a community, you are likely connected to people who:

- Share a set of LGBTQ-affirming values

- Attend similar events or frequent similar spaces

- Understand what supports or threatens your resilience as an LGBTQ person

- Connect in a variety of ways, like online or in person

- Seek to understand and support other LGBTQ people

- Advocate for LGBTQ-affirming environments

- Feel there is something larger than their own individual identity as an LGBTQ person

Having community is important for your resilience as an LGBTQ person, whether you are an introvert or an extrovert. Many trans people who are introverts, for example, may connect with other queer and trans community members online. This is where they may feel the most support as they are exploring their identity. Queer and trans people of color who struggle to find support in their own local communities can connect with online LGBTQ communities of color. For others, it is important to connect in person as a community. In Chapter 8, you will think more about both in-person and online support groups and consider which you might prefer; here our discussion is about *having community* as an important part of resilience. Support groups and other supportive spaces can be a part of having community, but in this section you will build on the steps you used to explore your friendship-making patterns to understand how to build a community that increases your resilience. Anushka Aqil credits her community for much of her resilience as a queer person in a university graduate program.

As student who has been in the university for many years, I notice I occupy two main communities—one by default and one chosen with extreme intent. Within my ivory tower community, every day is a struggle to ensure that marginalized voices are heard, that White supremacy is consistently called out, and that work isn't done on communities but with communities. At the end of every day, I am fortunate to have my chosen community to lean upon, learn from, and grow with through critical self-reflection and constant reimagining of what our queer futures can look like. My survival and my work to uplift the voices of the communities is because I have community that holds me accountable and affords me safety—it is only because of them that I can go beyond surviving and begin thriving as a queer and South Asian American person.

—Anushka Aqil, South Asian, queer, cisgender
woman, student activist

In the next resilience practice, you'll reflect on what you want in a community that supports your resilience as an LGBTQ person.

RESILIENCE PRACTICE: Making the Best Community for You

In this resilience practice, you get to dream up the community you would like to have. Think about each prompt and respond.

What types of communities are you a part of right now?

_____

_____

_____

_____

As an LGBTQ person, what types of community would you like to have?

_____

_____

_____

_____

What would you need to do to build connection with your community?

_____

_____

_____

_____

Based on the preceding prompt, list three specific next steps you can take to further develop a community that supports your resilience as an LGBTQ person.

_____

_____

_____

_____

_____

_____

What was it like to reflect on the type of community that would encourage and support your resilience? Did you realize you have certain preferences or needs as you develop this community? Take a moment to think about when you can implement your three next steps. Don't rush yourself, but consider when you could take action.

Resilience Wrap-Up

In this chapter you've learned how important relationships and community are to your mental health and well-being as an LGBTQ person. You also explored that neither of these endeavors will happen overnight; rather, you need to engage in steps along the way. Developing relationships and community building is a process. Here are a few things to remember:

- It's important to know that your mental health and well-being are intricately linked to the health of your relationships.

- Experiencing LGBTQ discrimination makes strong relationship skills even more important, so you have meaningful support when you need it most.

- There is a range of different types of relationships, so it's helpful to occasionally take an inventory of the types of relationships in your life; then you'll know which types you would like to develop.

- Our cultural values and upbringing inform how we develop healthy relationships. You get to choose which cultural values increase your resilience as an LGBTQ person, and which values decrease it.

- Developing friendships is a part of building community.

- By knowing your boundaries and communicating your boundaries to others, you can deepen and maintain important friendships.

- It is helpful to consider what type of community you would like to feel a part of, with special consideration of how much this community might add to or subtract from your resilience.

In Chapter 8, you'll move from growing your resilience through developing relationships and building community to how to get LGBTQ support and resources you need to help your resilience grow as a queer or trans person.

Getting Support and Knowing Your Resources

In the preceding chapters you have explored resilience based on your gender and sexual orientation and other identities, as well as how to be resilient to negative messages about being LGBTQ and knowing your self-worth as a queer or trans person. Because the lives and achievements of LGBTQ people are not embedded in school curricula or learned about in family and other informal social settings, you may know very little about your own LGBTQ community and may have few LGBTQ-affirming resources. Part of building your resilience as an LGBTQ person is knowing the important practice of getting support and having LGBTQ-affirming resources that you can rely on during tough times.

This important practice includes knowing when you need help and how to ask for it. It also includes being able to sift through resources to determine how LGBTQ-affirming they are. You learn more about when you do and do not need support as a queer or trans person. You also learn more about the type of support you need. It then becomes easier to develop healthy practices of relying on people and other resources you truly need to build your resilience. In this chapter, I'll help you figure out which types of support work best for you, based on your life and your personality, and how LGBTQ community events may be an important part of your resilience.

The Role of Support in Sustaining Resilience

Think for a moment. When was the last time you really needed support? Were you mildly stressed, or was it a major event that led to your needing support? Did you talk to someone about needing support, or did you decide to go it alone because you thought no one would understand what you were going through? These questions should get you thinking about whether supportive community and resources are an important part of your life, how much you have accessed them, and even how much you have received support that is *actually supportive*. Many times you may not have had access as an LGBTQ person to the support you really did need, whether in your family, school, work, community, or other settings. Think of both the instances when you needed support and did not receive it, and when you did receive the needed support. The following resilience practice will help you identify your support experiences as you were growing up, as well as the types of support that feel most helpful to you.

Fall seven times, stand up eight.

—Japanese proverb

RESILIENCE PRACTICE: Reflecting on What You've Learned about Receiving Support

Your family can be like a mini-schoolhouse of learning, with your parents or caregivers serving as your caregivers, instructors, and authors of the textbooks! Whether you had great, middling, or poor relationships with your parents while growing up, you tend to observe and soak up how they exhibited their need for support, accepted support, refused support, or even pretended they did not need support. Consider these questions and write your responses:

What type of support did you see people receiving when you were growing up?

_____

_____

_____

_____

How do you remember people responding to giving or receiving this support?

_____

_____

_____

_____

Did you receive support or not as an LGBTQ person growing up?

_____

_____

_____

_____

If you did receive support as an LGBTQ person growing up, was it helpful, not helpful, or somewhere in between? If you didn't receive support, what was the support you needed?

_____

_____

_____

_____

What did you notice about your answers? Was it easy to think of examples of people receiving support when you were growing up, or was it more tough to remember? Was it easier to remember how people in your family responded to receiving support? Did it get more emotional or difficult to think about the support you needed, but may or may not have received, as a queer or trans person growing up? Your answers do not have to be precise, but you should get a sense for how much your family demonstrated that receiving support was important, and you should be starting to think about how your resilience as an LGBTQ person was affected by the support you did or did not receive.

Read what Sand Chang says about their resilience and how they make sure they are conscious of how to recharge, renew, and keep an eye on how to keep their resilience strong.

Resilience is a practice rather than something that I simply have as a trait or character asset. It's everything I do that fortifies me in a world that does not affirm all my identities all the time. What I need might change from day to day. There are times when a hard workout or doing yoga is what I need the most to ground myself in my body and detox from negativity [of] the external world, and there are times when I just need stillness. It might look like saying "no" to being in environments that I know will create more emotional labor for me. It might mean surrounding myself with supportive, loving people, or it might mean going inward and cultivating connection with myself or my spiritual practices. Around me I see how easy it is to check out, to numb, or dissociate through the trauma of everyday life. I certainly have done my share of that. Today I make every effort to make conscious choices toward long-term solutions rather than instant gratification or the illusion of being able to "fix" myself, others, or the world in a moment. For the most part, resilience is about choice or at least slowing down so that I have choices.

—Sand Chang, Chinese American,
genderqueer therapist

RESILIENCE PRACTICE: Identifying Which Sources of Support Work Well for You

Now that you have a general impression of how support was treated when you were growing up, let's talk about what support can look like, in a practical sense, and identify which sources of support you find most helpful.

Read through the listed sources of support, then in the left colum rate *how supportive* each seems to you, using a scale of 1 to 3, where 1 is very supportive, 2 is kind of supportive, and 3 is not supportive at all. Don't think about it too much—this is meant as a quick assessment of what you tend to respond to the most:

Rating	Sources of Support	Current Access
	Talking on the phone	
	Videoconferencing (like Skype, FaceTime)	
	Meeting someone in person	
	Spending time alone	
	Spending time with one other person	
	Connecting with a friend	
	Connecting with a family member	

	Going to a counselor or therapist	
	Receiving a pep talk	
	Processing what happened	
	Being reminded that you are a good person	
	Making a list or plan of what to do next	
	Feeling that someone is listening to you	
	Journaling	

Read through your list when you are done. As you look back over the list, take three different highlighter colors and use one each to highlight the sources of support you marked 1, 2, or 3. Then look at each of these three groupings and think about how much these are present in your life right now. Place a checkmark in the right column for those that you have access to right now.

This is just an initial assessment of where you are currently with receiving support. When you take time to reflect on this, you can gauge how much access you have to support. Next, we'll talk about the type of support you need related to your personality.

Knowing Your Personality and What Support Works Best for You

So far, you have reflected on how family influences can affect how you receive support, and you have explored the types of support that actually feel helpful to you. Your personality can play a large role in receiving support as well. We each have our own unique personality, but there are some common facets. For example, one major facet of personality is how *introverted* or *extroverted* you are.

Your degree of introversion and extroversion (most of us are somewhere on the continuum) plays a big role in the type of support you prefer. Introverts tend to want to be alone and work things out in their own head before they talk to someone else. Researching websites, reading books, or journaling are activities many introverts find helpful to settle their minds and get support. Being an introvert doesn't mean you don't like people or have difficulty receiving support from others. It just means that you tend to build your energy by being alone or with one other person, and you find this more helpful than hanging out with a lot of people or getting "cheered up."

On the other hand, extroverts tend to process their stress by being with others and may find going to a gathering or party is a helpful source of support (which could be a nightmare for an extreme introvert!). If you are extroverted, you get much of your energy from other people, so being around others is your natural tendency and can feel very supportive.

This isn't black or white; rather, think of extroversion and introversion as two ends of a continuum. You tend to have *preferences* in this facet of your personality, so you gravitate to a part of the continuum that is most comfortable to you. It may be that you find yourself toward the middle: sometimes feeling extroverted, so connecting with others will feel supportive, and other times feeling introverted, so spending time alone will be more helpful in building your internal energy and resources. Take a look at the continuum and think about where you might fall on it:

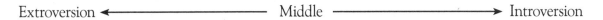

Extroversion ◀──────────────── Middle ────────────────▶ Introversion

Navigating Stress

No matter what type of stress you are facing, it is important to *not force yourself* to receive support that does not work for you. That is why this introversion-extroversion continuum is important. As an LGBTQ person, there is the everyday stress you can feel just from life in general. Then there is the stress that we discussed in the introduction, from having to navigate queer and trans stigma in society. Both types of stress—everyday stress and minority stress—can knock you off your center.

Now, when you are not under immediate stress, is when it can be helpful to attempt to *grow* the ways you can receive help. That is another reason knowing where you fall along this continuum can be important. If you tend toward one side, growing those support resources can help you. Some people think that being in the middle of the continuum is the most healthy position, as then you can more readily access both types of support. Regardless, it can be helpful to strengthen your ways of accessing support that are not your typical go-to's. This is especially important because LGBTQ people experience social stress on top of everyday types of stress, so they need a wider range of support.

LGBTQ-Specific Stress

As explored in earlier chapters, in the course of their lives queer and trans people experience some common sources of stress. Taking a closer look at some of these sources of stress can help shine a light on resources you can use to move through these experiences and get the support you need. Some instances of LGBTQ-specific stress are more intense than others, so they can require different types of help. Getting verbally harassed as an LGBTQ person is terrible, and if you are alone when it happens it can feel even more scary. Some queer and trans people, especially people of color, may not trust the police as a potential source of help because of the long history of negative experiences LGBTQ communities of color have had with the police. So they may turn to community members for help before they turn to the police. In addition, emotional, physical, sexual, and spiritual abuse can feel really different to different people. Likewise, reactions to rejection by family and friends—a common experience for queer and trans people—can differ depending on the type of relationship.

In addition to the stress of being different, there are different categories of LGBTQ-specific stress: intrapersonal, interpersonal, and institutional.

INTRAPERSONAL STRESS

You may have internalized negative thoughts about being LGBTQ (which we explored in Chapter 3), which may lead to feeling depressed, anxious, or even having suicidal thoughts, self-injuring, or abusing substances to cope with this stress. These internal types of stress fall into the category of *intrapersonal* LGBTQ-specific stress.

INTERPERSONAL STRESS

When you experience LGBTQ stigma in relationships with others in your family, social groups, school, work, or other settings, this is *interpersonal* LGBTQ-specific stress. When you experience interpersonal stress as a queer or trans person, you are being negatively targeted in some way about your identities. This targeting can be conscious, such as name-calling, or unconscious, such as someone assuming that you are straight or cisgender. Examples include being called an LGBTQ epithet while you are walking to meet a friend, hearing your supervisor make heterosexist remarks, being told you aren't a "real woman" if you are trans, or being kicked out of your home as an LGBTQ youth.

INSTITUTIONAL STRESS

Institutional LGBTQ-specific stress also can occur across a variety of settings and entail interacting with people, but it specifically includes systemic oppression and discrimination experienced when interacting with large systems. Examples include school and university systems, religious/spiritual institutions, and healthcare systems. Within these systems, there may be an explicit lack of rights for LGBTQ people, such as statutes in certain states allowing discrimination against queer and trans people and denial of services. There are also systems that are designed to serve straight people but not prepared to best serve LGBTQ people. For example, across the United States the laws that govern adopting or fostering children differ from state to state and often allow discrimination against LGBTQ people.

With institutional stress, it may be difficult to identify a single person or even a group of people as the source. The healthcare system, in which trans-related medical services aren't always guaranteed, is a key example of such institutional LGBTQ-specific stress.

The next resilience practice will help you identify the specific support you need when you experience LGBTQ-specific stress in interpersonal relationships or when interacting with institutional systems.

RESILIENCE PRACTICE: Do You Know What Support You Need When You Experience LGBTQ-Specific Stress?

The goal of this resilience practice is to consider common sources of LGBTQ-specific stress that you may have experienced, or could experience, and see whether you feel prepared in knowing what steps to take in response. The sample list covers the three categories of LGBTQ-specific stress we just discussed: intrapersonal, interpersonal, and institutional. For each item:

- If you have experienced that LGBTQ-specific stress, place a checkmark to the *left*.

- If you know the support and resources you would need to cope with this LGBTQ-specific stress, place a checkmark to the *right*.

For each category there are additional blank lines where you can add any LGBTQ-specific stress experiences not listed.

Intrapersonal

Have Experienced	LGBTQ-Specific Stress	Have Support and Resources
	Feeling depressed about being LGBTQ	
	Feeling anxious that someone may find out you are LGBTQ	
	Having suicidal thoughts because you are LGBTQ	
	Cutting or injuring yourself because you are LGBTQ	
	Wishing you were not LGBTQ	
	Abusing substances, like alcohol or drugs	
	Engaging in unsafe sex	
	Wishing you were not LGBTQ	

Interpersonal

Have Experienced	LGBTQ-Specific Stress	Have Support and Resources
	Being rejected by a family member or friends	
	Being called an LGBTQ epithet	
	Hearing a teacher make a heterosexist remark	
	Not being invited to work events your colleagues attend	
	Hearing from a religious/spiritual leader that you will "go to hell"	
	Experiencing emotional, physical, sexual, or spiritual abuse	

Institutional

Have Experienced	LGBTQ-Specific Stress	Have Support and Resources
	Not being able to access important health care safely	
	Feeling unsafe at school or work	
	Experiencing legal stress	
	Experiencing political stress related to anti-LGBTQ sentiment	
	Feeling scared to use public facilities, like restrooms	
	Not being able to access safe housing	
	Being afraid of being stopped by the police	

Important note: If you checked that you are feeling suicidal, it is important to call an LGBTQ-affirmative hotline immediately. A good resource is The Trevor Project (http://www.thetrevor project.org; 1-866-488-7386); you can also visit your local hospital emergency room. Because LGBTQ communities have high rates of suicidality, it is important to get help immediately if you are having thoughts of hurting yourself or have a plan or the means to hurt yourself. Talking about suicide will not make it happen, but *not* talking about suicidal feelings can place you in great danger of isolation and a lack of support.

You have explored some difficult situations in this book, and completing this list may feel very difficult, because some LGBTQ-specific stress, when it is chronic or situational, can also be traumatic over time. In addition, some categories of LGBTQ stress include such harmful experiences that you may begin wanting to hurt yourself in some way. Notice which LGBTQ-specific stresses you checked on the left but not on the right—indicating you experience this stress, but lack resources to deal with it. If you didn't know what might help you to cope with some of the scenarios in this exercise, don't worry; the rest of the chapter is devoted to helping you find those resources. You should end the chapter feeling more confident to check more items on the right. In Chapter 5, you learned about standing up for yourself; in this chapter you are learning about building your own resources and creating community that supports you as a queer or trans person.

Accessing Stable Structures for LGBTQ Support

Now let's think about more specific types of support, other than family or friends, which can help you manage and heal from LGBTQ-specific stress. Friends and family members who are LGBTQ-affirming, and also colleagues and peers in work and school settings, can be important sources of support. However, sometimes these sources are unstable or difficult to rely on when you need help the most. Other times you may lack access to supportive people in these categories. In the next sections, you will read about additional sources of LGBTQ support that may make sense for you.

Our wounds are often the openings into the best and most beautiful part of us.

—David Richo, White, cisgender, straight, author

Counseling

Counseling, also called therapy, can be an important way to find support just for you. Even when you have some support as a queer or trans person from people in your community, it can be helpful to have a space and a person solely dedicated to your own healing. Because microaggressions and macroaggressions can add up over time, creating more risk and vulnerability in your life, counseling can be a good way to check in and see how you are doing as an

LGBTQ person and what you need to be resilient and thrive. Through counseling you can not only learn more about yourself but also work with your counselor to proactively heal from LGBTQ stigma you may have experienced or internalized.

You may feel that counseling isn't for you. Some research has found that some groups, like people of color or immigrants, may not feel as comfortable as other groups in accessing counseling (Sue & Sue, 2015). (I'll discuss community indigenous sources of support later in this chapter.) Even if you do feel that counseling is right for you in terms of support, it can be difficult to find an LGBTQ-affirming counselor. To ensure that you work with a good counselor, look for one with these qualifications and experience:

- License as a counselor, social worker, school counselor, psychologist, psychiatrist, or nurse practitioner

- Understanding of LGBTQ concerns, so you do not have to teach them about queer or trans education and competence

- A record of advocacy for LGBTQ and ability to help you move through LGBTQ barriers in society, such as writing a letter for referral to trans medical services

- Empowerment perspective on working with LGBTQ people and, if they are a cisgender or straight person, awareness of their privilege

- Familiarity with queer and trans communities in your city and state

- Completion of continuing education on LGBTQ concerns in mental health, and commitment to ongoing education.

Finding a counselor can be challenging, as some counselors will list LGBTQ concerns as a specialty but actually engage in *conversion therapy*. Conversion therapy is an unethical approach to counseling, wherein the counselor attempts to guide or pressure the person to change their gender or sexual orientation. These approaches are unethical because rather than supporting or improving the client's mental health, they harm it, according to research. Your counselor's professional ethics require that they respect and support you for who you are in terms of your sexual orientation and gender identity—not impose on you their religious and/or societal beliefs that conflict with who you know yourself to be. Other challenges may arise when seeking a counselor, such as whether you have insurance, live in a rural area with limited options, live in an LGBTQ-negative community, or are not employed. If you do not have insurance or are not employed, it is helpful to search for a pro-bono or reduced-fee (sliding scale) counselor. If you are in a rural or LGBTQ-negative environment, look for counselors who work online (called tele-counseling).

Support and Counseling Groups

Many LGBTQ people find participating in a support group immensely helpful. Support groups can center on queer or trans issues, or may include all LGBTQ identities within one support group. Support group facilitators typically may not have formal mental health training, whereas counseling groups tend to be led by mental health professionals. There are advantages and disadvantages to each, depending on your needs for support at any given time. Some counseling groups run for a certain period (like a six-week, eight-week, or twelve-week group) that you must sign up for and pay for in advance, whereas support groups tend to be free and allow attendees to drop in as they need to for support. Both counseling groups and support groups can also "meet" online, not just in person. For both types of groups, there is a wide range of leadership and membership possibilities, so just as you need to ask some important questions when seeking a counselor, you need to ask similar questions about group leaders and members:

- What is the purpose of the group—support, counseling, or educational?

- Who leads the group, and what is their background and training?

- Who are the typical members of the group?

- Is there an expected commitment level for group attendance?

These questions can be really important in relation to where LGBTQ group members are with their identity development and self-definition. For instance, trans support groups can vary widely between members who are more focused on accessing medical interventions and supporting one another in this, and those who value gender fluidity and reflect on general experiences in society rather than primarily on medical treatment. Before you join a particular group, talk to current or recent members in person and online—like in email and on social media—about their experiences there. The "current or recent" part is important, as changes in group membership can influence the group's purpose and content.

Community Resources

Whereas individual counseling, group counseling, and support groups tend to be ongoing, sometimes you might need a different type of support that is not on a regular weekly schedule, such as community resources and events. Community resources can include a range of queer and trans organizations (local, state, regional, national, international) that are either brick-and-mortar organizations, online organizations, or other types of community groups. Many of these spring up as community needs arise. For instance, when anti-LGBTQ legislation is proposed, often organizations begin working locally to educate voters and work to prevent passage. When anti-trans bathroom laws started appearing in state legislatures across the country, various community groups came together to collaborate and resist this oppressive legislation.

Why do these types of groups matter to all queer and trans people? Because these groups typically have the most up-to-date and current resources related to LGBTQ civil rights. During times that anti-LGBTQ social sentiment is fomented and increases, such a resource can explicitly inform you of your bathroom rights in a school, college campus, or public setting. Knowing your specific rights can become more important at different times in your life. For instance, if your partner is hospitalized or if you are adopting, knowing which organizations work on these areas of LGBTQ civil rights can not only help you be resilient during a tough time, but also increase your resilience through stronger connections to LGBTQ-empowering resources. Complete the next resilience practice to identify LGBTQ community resources you can access when you need them.

RESILIENCE PRACTICE: Mapping Your LGBTQ Community Resources

In this practice, you'll explore how much you know about your LGBTQ community resources at the local, state, regional, national, and international levels. Check the statements below for which you can affirm that you know how to access the appropriate resources as a queer or trans person that empower you and support your civil rights.

I am aware of organizations that:

- ☐ Support LGBTQ people of my generation, such as children, adolescents, young adults, adults in midlife, and older adults

- ☐ Compile information related to LGBTQ health care

- ☐ Support LGBTQ biological, adoptive, and foster parents

- ☐ Gather information on LGBTQ legal rights, like marriage and the tax code

- ☐ Compile information on LGBTQ rights in housing and other neighborhood concerns

- ☐ Gather information on LGBTQ interactions with the police and other legal enforcement

- ☐ Track information on legislation impacting LGBTQ people

☐ Compile information on LGBTQ hate crimes

☐ Track information on LGBTQ international concerns

What do you notice? Do you have more information about some sorts of organizational resources than about others? Rounding out your knowledge in any areas where it's lacking will help you not only access support for yourself when you need it, but also support others in your community, whether or not they share similar identities with you.

Community Events

In some ways, community events dovetail with community resources. These events can pop up as LGBTQ needs arise, or they may be established traditions to address long-term needs in the queer and trans community. For instance, the Trans Day of Remembrance is a long-standing tradition held around the world on November 20 to honor the lives of trans people who have died related to anti-trans bias. Queer and Trans Pride events are also long-standing events, but these can signal a different tone for communities as a reminder of the unique and important contributions of LGBTQ people that should be celebrated. Here are some other notable queer and trans events:

• Trans Day of Remembrance

• Trans Day of Resilience

• Day of Silence

• Stonewall Riots Anniversary

• Awareness Weeks for individual groups within the LGBTQ community

• World AIDS Day

• National Coming Out Day

• LGBT History Month

• Racial/Ethnic Pride celebrations, such as Black Pride, Latinx Pride

Are these common events in your city or cities nearby? Were there some events you did not know about or recognize? Google the events you were not as familiar with, and know that many LGBTQ events are also held online for those who may not be able to travel to these community occasions. Kirk Surgeon's story speaks to the importance of community connections and events in fostering resilience in his life.

Coming out for me has been an ongoing process of self-realization. The first time I really came out was to myself. Once I came to the realization that I was not straight, I delved into information from the public library, alternative newspapers, and magazines on gay culture (this was the pre-Google era, LOL!). From those sources, I discovered and connected with the Triangle Community Center (TCC) in Norwalk, Connecticut, which was close to where I then lived. I didn't realize, at the time, how fortunate I was to have ready access to a gay community center close by that provided affirming support and services to me on my coming-out journey. TCC helped me to see the power of cooperation in empowering the LGBTQI [Lesbian, Gay, Bisexual, Transgender, Queer or Questioning, and Intersex] community. There I was able to meet with individuals who were also just coming out as well as those who were well on their own journey. Both groups of individuals provided me with invaluable lessons on how to navigate being gay in Connecticut and New York, as I didn't realize how much I didn't know about gay life. As I learn more about myself I realize the truth in the statement information is power and liberation. The most important lesson I learned was that I was not the only one! I was not the only one who didn't know where to go to meet gay friends. I was not the only one afraid of what my parents would do when I came out to them. I was not the only one who was scared of what being gay would mean to my friends, my career, my extended family. I was not as alone in my feelings and doubts as I had thought. I was not alone, as I was a part of a community that I could embrace and which would embrace me if I would be brave enough to willingly be a part of that community. I'm glad I chose to embrace that part of me and the community that came with being gay, as that community has been one of my greatest supports.

—Kirk Surgeon, African American, gay, cisgender, community organizer

Religious or Spiritual Support

For many queer and trans people, religious and/or spiritual support is an integral aspect of their lives. For some, it is also a double-edged sword. On the one hand, their religious and/or spiritual beliefs help them move through hard times and are a critical component of resilience. On the other hand, many of these same people have been hurt by religious and/or spiritual groups because of their gender or sexual orientation. Not all people identify religion or spirituality as an important part of their resilience, as some identify as atheist or agnostic. However, even for people in those categories, religious and spiritual traditions can be frightening and sometimes even dangerous, as some leaders in these traditions preach against queer and trans communities. For instance, I identify as a Sikh (a South Asian religion). Even though I did not grow up with a religious concept of being a sinner, I grew up in the very Catholic city of New Orleans, where these were common beliefs and messages that my fellow queer and trans peers were exposed to as they worshipped. My atheist and agnostic friends who were raised in religious or spiritual homes had similar experiences, and these negative self-beliefs were internalized. The next resilience practice will help you see how religious/spiritual belief systems may have been helpful, harmful, or a combination of both for you as a queer or trans person.

RESILIENCE PRACTICE: Religious and/or Spiritual Resources as Supports, Barriers, or Both

In this practice, you'll explore how religious or spiritual belief systems have influenced how you view yourself as a queer or trans person. Reflect on your life thus far, and answer the following questions. Note: You do not have to subscribe to a certain religious and/or spiritual belief to move through this resilience practice activity.

Was religion and/or spirituality a large part of your upbringing?

_____

_____

_____

_____

Was religion and/or spirituality helpful, harmful, or a combination in learning to affirm your gender and sexual orientation?

_____

_____

_____

_____

Right now, is religion and/or spirituality helpful, harmful, or both as a resource that helps you feel good as a queer or trans person?

_____

_____

_____

_____

If you could go back in time and talk to your younger self about how religious and/or spiritual approaches should support queer and trans communities, what would you say?

_____

_____

_____

_____

If you were asked to talk to religious and/or spiritual leaders about what you think they should do to support queer and trans people in their resilience, what would you say?

_____

_____

_____

_____

La cultura cura. (Culture heals.)

—José Antonio Burciaga, Chicano, cisgender,
straight, author

Indigenous Healing and Support Systems

The word "indigenous" refers to cultural ways of healing that are important resources to many communities. These cultural ways of healing may be integral resources you grew up with or were introduced to along the way. Some, but not all, indigenous models of healing may be related to religious and/or spiritual supports. Growing up, I was introduced to ayurvedic medicine (Indian holistic approaches) as part of my culture. This indigenous healing resource, thought to be thousands of years old, relies on various natural treatments, like food or herbal remedies, to relieve stress and tension. East Asian indigenous approaches such as traditional Chinese medicine (TCM) have a similar approach, whereby personal experiences of pain are related to imbalances in the individual's energy field. Native American indigenous approaches view an individual's experience of stress as related to nature and the larger world, which can aid in healing.

These are just a few examples of indigenous healing, and in the U.S. culture all are still generally viewed as not mainstream (with a few exceptions, such as acupuncture). However, these healing resources are considered very much mainstream within their cultures of origin. Many queer and trans people find that as they recover their sense of self-worth and validation of their identities, they can begin to also explore and embrace alternatives to mainstream Western healing such as counseling or psychiatric medicine. This is not to say one approach is more helpful than the other, only that it is important to acknowledge multiple modes of healing resources with a long history of use that can help queer and trans people increase their resilience.

Other Types of Support: Considering Our Multiple Identities

In Chapter 2, you learned the significance of all of our social identities within the queer and trans community, such as racial/ethnic identity or disability identity. This significance can be really important when it comes to the type of support and resources you need to be resilient in the world as an LGBTQ person.

As with some of the other areas of support, our need for these resources may change over time. For example, during one period of my life, I really needed to be connected with a South Asian queer and trans group. Within this supportive space, I could connect with people who grew up with similar traditional foods, holidays, dance, music, and culture. I literally felt at home in these groups, which really increased my resilience. As a reminder, here are *some* examples of different social identities—there are many more, but this is a good start to get you remembering parts of your identity in addition to your gender and sexual orientation:

- Race/ethnicity
- Class
- Disability

- Migration status, such as immigrant, refugee, asylee, undocumented

- Education level, such as high school, college, or graduate school

- Neighborhood setting, such as urban, suburban, or rural

- Political affiliation, such as Democratic, Progressive, Radical, Republican, and Libertarian

- Religious and/or spiritual affiliation

RESILIENCE PRACTICE: Other Types of Support: What Did You Need Then, and What Do You Need Now?

This resilience practice will help you explore your current needs for support and resources related to different aspects of your identity. Consider these questions and respond.

When you were growing up, what types of supportive spaces related to your social identities did you need? Were you able to access these spaces?

_____

_____

_____

_____

Currently, what types of supportive spaces related to your social identities do you need? Have you been able to access these spaces?

_____

_____

_____

_____

Are there types of support spaces related to your social identities that you prefer not to access at this time?

_____

_____

_____

_____

Your responses should give you an idea of whether there are specific subgroups within the LGBTQ community that have been—or would be—helpful for you to access as resources. Remember, there is no "right" answer to these questions; there is only what is true for you at this moment. And that truth can change, depending on what is going on in terms of current events, noticing your changing needs, and influences from your community. For example, after 9/11, there was a lot of targeting of the South Asian community in the United States. At that time I reconnected with a South Asian queer and trans group, as well as other more general and broad South Asian–serving organizational supports.

Read how Roan Coughtry builds community as a key component of their resilience, and how building community is an intentional act for them to grow their resilience.

Building community is an important source of resilience, both personally and collectively. For myself, simply being around people who reflect all sorts of gender possibilities—Who see and value my gender without question or confusion—was so healing in my coming-out process and continues to be today. Being able to build family and love with people in queer creative ways validates my desires and longings. On a collective level, building community with one another—through queered relationships, queered families, witnessing each others' magic, and mutual support—quite literally keeps us alive, and it also helps us expand and thrive. So much in society fosters this "divide and conquer" strategy that's meant to keep us apart, keeps us isolated, encourages us to turn on each other and fight our own, rather than noticing the real systems that oppress and exploit. Resilience requires that we work through this and build community in spite of this—both within queer circles and expanding beyond them. Our power is in community, in partnerships, in brilliant collaborations and fierce love.

—Roan Coughtry, White, poly, genderqueer,
sex positive community organizer

RESILIENCE PRACTICE: What Current LGBTQ-Affirming Resources Can You Access?

Now that you've looked at different types of resources you can access, you're in a position to reflect on what sorts of support would be useful for you *right now*. Check off the sources of interpersonal support that you think would be helpful for you to access right now or in the future. There are some extra spaces in case you would like to get more specific about what local LGBTQ-affirming resources would fit your needs for support:

☐ LGBTQ-affirming individual counseling

☐ LGBTQ-affirming counseling group or support group

☐ LGBTQ-affirming community resource or event

☐ LGBTQ-affirming religious or spiritual community

☐ Indigenous healing

☐ Support related to your other identities

☐ _____

☐ _____

☐ _____

☐ _____

What did you notice as you checked off the list? Do these next steps seem doable? And who could help you along the way in accessing these supports? Were the supports you checked off more related to being LGBTQ, or more about your other identities? Your resilience is intrinsically linked to the supports you have in your life, so taking time to reflect on what you need and identifying the very next step is an important way to grow your resilience.

Resilience Wrap-Up

You build resilience step by step, through learning more about yourself and the world around you. As I have talked about in this chapter, you experienced different types of support growing up; you had needs that either were addressed or went unaddressed. Finding the best support for you as an LGBTQ person is an ongoing process. For example, during some periods of my life, being part of a queer and trans-specific space was important to me as a genderqueer person. In these spaces, I could express my gender exploration as it was happening in the moment without any judgment. At other times, I did not need queer or trans space at all, as I felt more integrated and solid in my identities. Other times, as I shared earlier, I needed other supports related to my racial/ethnic identity. Accessing support, however, can be influenced by a number of factors. Remember these pointers:

- You tend to learn about whether it is acceptable to receive support from your family and those you perceive as models while growing up.

- Your personality—for example, whether you're more introverted or extroverted—can influence the type of support you need.

- LGBTQ-specific stress is common, so it's important to know how and when to access support.

- If you begin feeling suicidal or like you want to self-harm, get help immediately (contact The Trevor Project, http://www.thetrevorproject.org; 1-866-488-7386).

- Supports and resources can come in the form of individual counseling, counseling and support groups, community resources and events, and indigenous healing, and within LGBTQ group spaces.

- Religious and/or spiritual traditions can be important supportive spaces for queer and trans people with those beliefs; those who identify as atheist or agnostic can also find support in those communities. However, there is a long history of people misusing religious and/or spiritual traditions in terms of anti-LGBTQ teachings.

In Chapter 9, you take everything you have learned so far—from knowing your multiple identities as an LGBTQ person, to knowing your self-worth and identifying affirming supports and resources, to exploring the resilience that you can develop when you experience hope about being LGBTQ—and seek and feel inspiration as a queer or trans person.

Getting Inspired

From reading earlier chapters, you know that resilience is natural. Just as when you break a bone, it heals stronger at the broken places, your resilience can strengthen over time. Getting inspired can take your resilience to an entirely new level. It is essential that you know how to bounce back from hard times as a queer or trans person, and inspiration can be the secret ingredient, reminding you how critical your resilience is to your well-being. In this chapter you will learn to prioritize being inspired, which includes learning new and different things about yourself that you may not have realized previously. From cultivating hope for the future, to the role of mentors, to identifying what you love to do, the resilience practices in this chapter help you explore how to plug into the inspiration that strengthens your resilience.

Building Hope as an Essential Resilience Resource

You know when you are feeling hopeful, right? Your mood is elevated, and you are filled with anticipation that something good is afoot! The *Merriam-Webster* dictionary defines hope as "a feeling of expectation and desire for a certain thing to happen." Feeling hopeful as a queer or trans person helps quell the threats to your resilience, as you have a strong idea or expectation that not only will something good happen, but you also deserve good things to happen in your life. So hope is connected to the self-worth and self-esteem that you learned about in Chapter 4. In the next resilience practice, you'll take a quick inventory of things you have been hopeful about as a queer or trans person.

RESILIENCE PRACTICE: What Does Hope Look Like in Your Life?

Think of some situations in which you have felt hopeful. In response to the questions, write about those experiences.

Describe a recent situation you felt hopeful about.

_____

_____

_____

How did you know you were feeling hopeful? Were there things you felt in your body (such as excitement, nervousness)?

_____

_____

_____

Did you let others know you were feeling hopeful, or did you keep it to yourself? What was it like sharing or not sharing that hopefulness?

_____

_____

_____

As you wrote about this experience of hope, did you notice that you also had some not-so-positive feelings as you experienced hope? For example, did you feel scared to be hopeful? Did you stop yourself from being hopeful? Respond to the following questions, and explore some of these experiences further.

What did you need to support your hopeful feelings in this situation?

_____

_____

_____

Did you trust or distrust your hopeful feelings in this situation?

_____

_____

_____

How did your feelings of trust or distrust influence your overall hopeful feelings?

_____

_____

_____

How was it for you, responding to this set of questions? When you feel hope, do you let yourself have that feeling? Or do you start distrusting that feeling? The feeling of hope can come with some nagging questions about whether you can trust in hope, and it may entail a little healthy anxiety, such as "Will I get this job that I want?" It is helpful to know how you typically interact with your feelings of hope because this can influence how resilient you feel in tough situations. Because LGBTQ people experience discrimination, it can be hard to trust when you are feeling hopeful about the future—which I will talk more about next.

Hope is being able to see that there is light despite all of the darkness.

—Archbishop Desmond Tutu, South African,
cisgender, straight male, human rights activist

Experiencing Hope as an LGBTQ Person

Hope is a pretty cool feeling, but as you learned in the preceding resilience practice, like every human being, you have your own personal patterns in how and why you let yourself feel hopeful. Hope can get kind of dicey for you as an LGBTQ person, because discrimination is real, and you shouldn't expect yourself or others to just hope your way out of it! Still, because hope has been shown to be a critical aspect of resilience for LGBTQ people (Singh, Hays, & Watson, 2011), it is important to cultivate it. Cultivating hope in this manner becomes like tending to a garden. There are the weeds (discrimination) growing in the garden of your resilience that need to be identified and plucked out so that your garden (yourself!) can flourish. And still, even as you create the most beautiful garden and use the highest-quality soil and diligent watering to nourish your garden, the wind (society) can still carry weed seeds right back into the middle of your enriched garden. Get the metaphor?

In this regard, as an LGBTQ person, you can think of hope not only as an experience that is an important aspect of your resilience, but also as a verb. Amid the windblown seedlings of anti-LGBTQ discrimination that threaten your own hope and self-growth, strengthening your wishes or hopes for certain things to happen in your life can help keep you on track toward living the life you truly want to live. So, hope as a verb entails that same expectation and positive outlook as when you are feeling hopeful, but it is specifically planted and cultivated.

Paying attention to hope as a verb in your life as a queer or trans person does imply some trust in the world, which can show you that the world will not always be fair. So, let's talk about that for a moment. A few years ago, Dan Savage—a well-known gay, cisgender Seattle journalist—famously began a campaign geared to supporting LGBTQ youth that he called "It Gets Better." His call to LGBTQ youth essentially was aimed at comforting them, asserting that they may have to deal with anti-LGBTQ oppression now, but it would get better as they became adults. Many queer and trans activists of color and White allies balked at this notion for several reasons: first, Savage was not reflecting on the White and male privilege that helped him "get better" as a gay, cisgender adult dealing with LGBTQ oppression; and second, there is an important role all people should play in supporting LGBTQ youth in *making* it better—not just hoping for things to get better.

I bring up this "It Gets Better" campaign specifically in our exploration of cultivating hope as a verb in building your resilience. This cultivation of hope is active—not passive. I do not want you to wait until things get better to grow your hope for your own dreams and thriving in the future. This cultivation of hope is grounded in the intersectionality of your identities that you explored in Chapter 2—issues of privilege and oppression can either support (privilege) or challenge (oppression) your development of hope as an LGBTQ person. It doesn't magically "get better" for everyone in the same ways, so the intersection of your identities really does matter and will shape your experience of growing your hope. This cultivation of hope is also mindful of anti-LGBTQ discrimination—it is important to develop hope despite the messages that you shouldn't feel good about your future at all.

This is a serious issue, actually. It may feel naïve to be hopeful about the world as an LGBTQ person, considering both how bad things can be for your community and the challenges you face individually. However, if you're not clear what this "getting better" should look or feel like (remind you of what you learned about boundary setting and self-worth as an LGBTQ person?), then you are stuck in the muck of "this is just the way it is going to be." That muck is where the LGBTQ community faces depression, anxiety, suicidality, substance abuse, and other serious concerns.

Many times in my own life, under the weight of racism and anti-LGBTQ messages, I just gave up on hope altogether. But what I was missing at the time was the self-worth to notice when I had lost both my hope and the support I needed to nourish my hope so it could grow. I 100 percent didn't need to be forced to feel hopeful or to act as if I was hopeful when I was not. That is not true hope. In short, we are not talking about the type of hope where other people hope things get better with anti-LGBTQ oppression. When you cultivate hope as a verb, you are telling yourself, "I am valuable enough to dream a future that I deserve." Hope then becomes a shield from discrimination and a reminder of the solidity of your expectations and dreams. Let's explore more of that in the next resilience practice.

RESILIENCE PRACTICE: Cultivating Hope as a Verb

In this resilience practice, you get to think about why hope, enacted as a verb, could matter to you as an LGBTQ person in a reliable way, to remind you of the value of who you are and your expectations for your life. Write your responses to the following questions:

What are the challenges to cultivating hope as an LGBTQ person?

_____

_____

_____

How do your multiple identities (like race/ethnicity, disability, class) influence how you cultivate hope?

_____

_____

_____

What are the opportunities for cultivating hope as an LGBTQ person?

_____

_____

_____

As an LGBTQ person, how can cultivating hope help you trust your own value more?

_____

_____

_____

As an LGBTQ person, what do you need in order to build hope in your life?

_____

_____

_____

List a few people with whom you can talk about building hope as an LGBTQ person in order to be more resilient.

_____

_____

_____

As you wrote your responses, did you notice common themes? When you explored your multiple identities related to building hope, did those themes change or become more specific? Was it easy to write about your needs for building hope? Sometimes asking for help with feeling hopeful about your life as an LGBTQ person can feel really vulnerable. That's why I recommend having these conversations about hope with the people you trust the most. They can help you have hope-as-a-verb to be more resilient. Next, let's talk about how the link between hope and inspiration can help you increase your resilience as an LGBTQ person.

Connecting Hope with Inspiration

Inspiration is the motivation you feel mentally and emotionally (and some might say spiritually) to create, innovate, and grow in unique ways. You may be thinking, "Wait; what does inspiration really have to do with resilience?" Well, this isn't the cheesy movie type of inspiration, where the main character overcomes all odds (although those types of movies can be fun to watch). Some people think inspiration is something that artists and other creative types feel every day in their work (which a lot of artists would likely say is rare). However, inspiration is important for you as an LGBTQ person, as you're likely finding new ways to express yourself and do things that are unique to you. Add a dose of LGBTQ discrimination, and you can see why inspiration is far from cheesy movieland. Read what Krista Jones shares about what inspires her resilience.

I draw most of my inspiration from the need for authentic self-expression, experience, and passion. I believe that embracing these deep-rooted needs has contributed to my resilience as both an artist and LGBTQ person. The need for authenticity has driven me to overcome many obstacles, including empowering myself and overcoming conditioned self-destructive behaviors. By persevering through gender and sexual identity challenges, I have gained self-love, compassion, and resilience in many other areas of my life. This has given me a more expansive understanding of my own value and self-worth as a person who identifies outside of society's "norm."

—Krista Jones, White, lesbian, cisgender, artist

Inspiration can also be the lifeblood that gets you excited and motivated to express your unique LGBTQ self in your personal and professional life in ways that feel true to you. I know I am feeling inspired when my heart soars and starts beating a little more quickly; often it is an emotional experience, and I may shed a few tears because I feel hopeful and moved about the world.

So you can see that inspiration and hope are inextricably linked. The more hope you cultivate, the more you can get inspired. The more inspired you are, the more hope you can experience and grow. In the next resilience practice, you'll explore what you think inspiration is.

RESILIENCE PRACTICE: Identifying the Best Sources of Inspiration for You

The goal of this resilience practice is to give you a quick feel for your take on inspiration. Complete the following sentence stems about inspiration, and as you do, notice the thoughts, feelings, and other reactions you may have. Keep your answers short—you'll come back to these ideas in a later practice and explore them further as they relate to your experience as an LGBTQ person:

Inspiration is _____.

When I hear the word "inspiration," I think of _____.

I feel most inspired when _____.

I feel least inspired when _____.

When I see others feeling inspired, I _____.

When others see me feeling inspired, they _____.

Was it easy for you to come up with a response? Or did you struggle to think of what to write? Are there any similarities in what kindles or deflates your inspiration? What did you notice when exploring how you experience others' inspiration and how others experience *your* inspiration? Some of what you allow yourself to experience with regard to inspiration depends on what you see or experience with others. Ultimately, to increase your resilience, you want to cultivate gratitude when you see others experiencing inspiration, as this reminds you of how nourishing inspiration is. Also, surrounding yourself with people who support you in getting inspired—rather than squelching your enthusiasm and excitement—contributes significantly to your overall resilience and well-being as an LGBTQ person. We'll be delving into that next.

Just don't give up trying to do what you really want to do. Where there is love and inspiration, I don't think you can go wrong.

—Ella Fitzgerald, African American, cisgender, singer

Learning What Inspires You as an LGBTQ Person

Now that you know what inspiration is and its connection to hope, the next step is thinking about what inspires you specifically as an LGBTQ person. Inspiration entails feeling motivated to be your unique self and express your own originality, while also potentially trying something new or taking a risk to do something you have always done one way, but tweaking it a bit or changing it altogether. Here are some things that inspire me as an LGBTQ person—see if some of them resonate with you:

- Listening to really good LGBTQ music that moves my soul. HOLYCHILD is my current fave

- Being around a sweet LGBTQ friend with whom I can experience exuberant, gut-busting laughter frequently

- Spending time in deep discussions about everything in the LGBTQ world with my partner

- Learning about LGBTQ cultures around the world and noticing how the United States is similar to or different from these cultures

- Participating in LGBTQ activism, community organizing, and freedom rights movements

- Writing poetry and writing in my journal

So getting inspired is really about identifying the sources of inspiration that motivate you to be curious about yourself and the world—and to potentially be willing to change (which you will explore more in Chapter 10).

Sometimes you need to take a departure from what you do to something that's slightly different in order to get inspiration.

—Tori Amos, cisgender, white, musician

Some of the resilience strategies we talked about in earlier chapters, such as having support (Chapter 8) and models of how to externalize negative LGBTQ messages (Chapter 3), are natural sources of inspiration. And other sources may be particularly important to you as an LGBTQ person. I like to use "who, what, where, when, how, and why" questions to remind me of my sources of inspiration, as used in the next resilience practice.

RESILIENCE PRACTICE: Identifying Your LGBTQ Sources of Inspiration

The goal of this resilience practice is to get you thinking about your inspirations as a queer or trans person. Respond to the following who, what, where, how, and why questions to identify these sources of inspiration:

Who inspires you to be your unique LGBTQ self?

_____

_____

_____

What inspires you to be your unique LGBTQ self?

_____

_____

_____

Where do you feel inspired to be your unique LGBTQ self?

_____

_____

_____

When are you inspired to be your unique LGBTQ self?

_____

_____

_____

How are you inspired to be your unique LGBTQ self?

_____

_____

_____

Why is it important to be inspired to be your unique LGBTQ self?

_____

_____

_____

As you completed your responses, you should have seen an emerging road map of sorts for not only what inspires you as an LGBTQ person, but also where the bumps in the road—or the potholes—may be in your sources of inspiration. The key to increasing your resilience is to find ways to further integrate the who, what, where, how, and why of your LGBTQ inspiration into your everyday life. This can be as simple as following an inspirational queer or trans person on social media, or posting a quotation that inspires you to be your unique and awesome LGBTQ self on a mirror in your bathroom or someplace you look often. Because you can't control the who, what, where, when, how, and why of anti-LGBTQ messages in society and discrimination, you need to be serious about building the things that inspire you as an LGBTQ person (but that doesn't mean it can't also be fun!).

Resilience Wrap-Up

In this chapter, you learned how getting inspired entails cultivating hope, and feeling inspiration about your unique self as an LGBTQ person increases your resilience:

- Developing your sense of hope for the future is an active process, not a passive one.

- Feeling hopeful about your life and cultivating your sense of hope does not mean you ignore anti-LGBTQ discrimination in the world. You just know how important your hope is in the face of a world that tries to take away your hope.

- Growing your hopefulness often entails having good support and doing a personal inventory of what expands or contracts your feelings of hope.

- Hope and inspiration are inextricably linked, so getting inspired means you feel more hopeful, and feeling more hopeful often entails being inspired.

- There are sources of general inspiration that can help you be more of your unique self, and there are sources of LGBTQ-specific inspiration that can help you value yourself more as a queer or trans person.

- Who, what, when, where, how, and why questions can help you quickly identify the strong and steady sources of inspiration in your life, and which sources you should cultivate further.

In Chapter 10, you'll move from developing your hope and inspiration personally as an LGBTQ person to learning how your resilience can be connected to making positive change in the world as a queer or trans person and giving back to your LGBTQ community.

Making Change and Giving Back

Just as getting inspired and feeling hopeful about your life goals and dreams increases your resilience, so does sharing your gifts and talents to help others. In this chapter, you'll explore how making positive social change and giving back to others can be an important part of your own resilience. As you have explored throughout this workbook, LGBTQ people face many life challenges. In the process of learning to be resilient to those challenges, queer and trans people end up learning a lot about themselves and the world. Practices in this chapter help you identify what gifts, talents, and/or skills you might want to share with people and communities of all sorts.

Helping Others Can Help You Increase Your Own Resilience

In my research on resilience, one interesting finding was consistent across racial/ethnic identity and age: it's all about helping others. This finding is interesting to me, because I don't think most people make this connection, whether they are queer or trans themselves or are strong LGBTQ allies. But when you think about it a little more deeply, it makes sense. Think about the last time you helped someone who was in need. You more than likely felt better about your ability to be helpful, and potentially you were rewarded by a thank-you or some expression of gratitude.

Well, science backs up the ways you can feel good when you help others (a practice commonly called altruism). When you help others, your brain releases endorphins. You feel good! As you feel good, this increases your feelings of gratitude for your ability to help others and for the gifts, talents, and skills you can share. Essentially, as your gratitude for the life you are living increases, when you are helping others you may feel like your problems are far away. In my research, the finding of helping others spanned a wide variety of helping—from working on specific social justice community causes, like efforts against animal cruelty and oppression, to helping out a friend or family member. I like to encourage and affirm others when they doubt themselves (no surprise that I'm writing this book, right?!), and I feel like it comes naturally to me. My South Asian cultural background and the gender socialization I had growing up likely have a lot to do with the ways I tend to help others. The following resilience practice will help you remember ways you have helped others and what it is like for you to be altruistic.

RESILIENCE PRACTICE: Identifying the Ways You Have Helped Others

The goal of this resilience practice is to help you recognize how you have helped other people and to explore the types of help you tend to give others. Remember, giving help to others does not have to be a grand notion of changing the world. It can be the everyday acts that you like sharing with others.

How do you feel about helping others?

_____

_____

_____

What strengths do you tend to use to help others?

_____

_____

_____

How are these strengths related to your multiple identities and cultural background?

_____

_____

_____

What responses do you tend to get from others when helping?

_____

_____

_____

As you responded to these questions, what did you notice? Were you surprised by how you felt about giving? Did giving to others feel like too much, or are you naturally drawn to helping others? What are the major ways you tend to help others? Did you feel excited, neutral, or unhappy responding to the questions?

No matter what you felt as you completed this resilience practice, there are limits to what you can give. Some people try to give beyond their limits, or have been taken advantage of because they were such ready helpers. Next, you will explore the natural limits to your giving. First, read how Ken Jackson has sought to help others and make positive social justice change in his community.

I work with the Georgia Safe Schools Coalition (GSSC), whose mission is to make schools safe for all students. Specifically, I serve on the board and do trainings throughout the state on supporting queer youth in schools. Also, I do consultations with families, youth, and schools on ways to create equitable environments for all students. As a counselor educator, I work with other educators to include authentic training for future counselors in their preparation programs and courses. As a practicing counselor in a school setting, I work with others to create policies, advocacy/educational opportunities, and counseling support for queer and trans youth and families. My work in this area allows for me to be a part in shaping a better world—even on a small level—and work to make schools better than they were than when I was a student. It gives me hope.

—Ken Jackson, White, cisgender, gay man,
school counselor

Your Resilience Limits When Helping Others

Because LGBTQ people have likely experienced a good deal of oppression in their life, you may feel there are some limits to what you can give. For instance, if you are feeling depressed or anxious, it can be all but impossible to even think about having the energy to give to others.

Or a particularly nasty anti-LGBTQ piece of legislation enacted in your state can reduce the energy you have to give. On the other hand, because altruism can give many people an energy boost and remind them of their gratitude for their own lives, sometimes even if you feel depressed or anxious, giving to others can help you remember the value of your own life. The key is to know the right amount of giving for *you*, based on your overall well-being, and to know when you are overdoing the giving at the expense of taking care of yourself.

In addition to the limited giving capacity you may feel as an LGBTQ person, you may be more introverted and prefer to give in ways that might feel small in the world. I encourage you to remember that no act of giving to others is too small! Again, the key is how that giving makes you feel. If the giving makes you feel drained afterward—or even just neutral—it may be time to reassess how you tend to give, to make sure you are within your boundaries for your overall well-being. Complete the next resilience practice to explore your limits when helping others.

RESILIENCE PRACTICE: Identifying the Ways You Have Helped Others

In this resilience practice, reflect on not only the ways you tend to give, but also on how you feel afterward.

How do you know you are giving too much when helping others?

_____

_____

_____

What thoughts and feelings do you have in these moments?

_____

_____

_____

What boundaries do you need to set in these instances?

_____

_____

_____

How can you use these boundaries to fine-tune your helping efforts, so you can give to others but preserve enough energy for yourself?

_____

_____

_____

Did you surprise yourself with any of your responses, or were they pretty much what you expected? As you explored your boundaries, did you think you tended to be within them, beyond them, or even unaware of your boundaries related to helping others? Which people in your life might make good accountability partners to check in with about helping others? There's one key question you can use to assess whether you've exceeded your boundaries: after helping others, do you feel more resilient or less resilient?

The best way to not feel hopeless is to get up and do something. Don't wait for good things to happen to you. If you go out and make some good things happen, you will fill the world with hope, you will fill yourself with hope.

—President Barack Obama, African American, multiracial, cisgender, straight male

How to Make the World a Better and Place: Community Organizing, Social Justice Activism, and Your Resilience

As I explored the research findings about how helping others can increase LGBTQ people's resilience, I found that much of it concerned community organizing and social justice activism. If you have not already gotten involved, I encourage you to explore this a bit. Even if you don't think community organizing and social justice activism are your cup of tea, it's helpful to look into it, because as queer and trans people we so typically experience anti-LGBTQ threats from the outside world.

What do I mean by community organizing and social justice activism? I think of community organizing as the efforts you can take to get involved in your community to bring about some sort of positive change. For instance, if LGBTQ youth do not have a support group they can attend, community organizing might entail raising some funds to pay a facilitator, or working with a local mental health agency to see what resources could be allocated to running this youth group. Community organizing can entail working with many stakeholders in the community—from lobbying government officials to working with community partner organizations and local residents. Read Suzann Lawry's story of how her resilience grew as she advocated against anti-LGBTQ policies and how her community change efforts were related to her identities as a lesbian and parent living in the South.

[For me] as a lesbian mother, the biggest catalyst for standing up for social justice was to protect my children who needed help navigating the questions that were coming at them on their playgrounds, in their classrooms, and inside their own skins; moreover, this was in 2003 in Georgia; they needed their family protected through equal access to marriage—now! So, I reached for wisdom about what to do from my relationships, because that's what Southern women do, and because the personal really is political. In hindsight, it was certainly an easier task to mobilize to "protect" my loved ones and to fight oppressive policies than it is now to really acknowledge how I continue to benefit [from] and perpetuate oppression on a daily basis. I could feel right, and worse, righteous; I didn't have to feel like a clumsy perpetual beginner. Ultimately, I believe it was inside those early efforts to "protect," studying strategies to effect change, and through those relationships and conversations, that I ended up stumbling upon my own evolving shared liberation. Stand up for social justice for the perfect reason, the imperfect reason, the selfish reason—the important act is to stand, and from there, your view will continue to change.

—Suzann Lawry, White, lesbian, cisgender woman, professor

I see social justice activism as very related to community organizing, but it can also entail more actions, such as street protests, marches, and rallies to call attention to an issue of inequity and injustice. For example, social justice activism might entail a protest at the local or state government office related to anti-LGBTQ legislation or lobbying public and private school officials to make school bathrooms trans-affirming. The combination of community organizing and social justice activism can be particularly powerful. I cofounded the Georgia Safe Schools Coalition to advocate for the rights of LGBTQ youth in schools, and the coalition was involved with many community partner organizations and members who engaged in a variety of activism related to policy change. The following resilience practice helps you reflect on how you feel about community organizing and social justice activism.

RESILIENCE PRACTICE: Taking Your Pulse about Community Organizing and Social Justice Activism

Community organizing and social justice activism vary widely, from small actions to big ones—from signing online petitions against LGBTQ discrimination and oppression of other sorts to marching in the streets. Think about the place of community organizing and social justice activism in your life.

When you think about community organizing and social justice activism, what thoughts and feelings come to mind?

_____

_____

_____

How have you engaged in community organizing and social justice activism previously?

_____

_____

_____

What motivates you to do community organizing and social justice activism—or deters you from doing it?

_____

_____

_____

Do you think community organizing and social justice activism increase your resilience, decrease your resilience, or both?

_____

_____

_____

Based on your responses, how would you describe your overall attitude toward community organizing and social justice activism? Have you been involved before and know your preferences and the efforts you support, or is this all new to you? Either way, in the next section you can further explore people's different roles in community organizing and social justice activism. We'll also shatter some of the myths about being involved in making social justice change.

What's Your Role in Community Organizing and Social Justice Change?

In the previous resilience practice you may have discovered that you want to get involved in making social justice change, but you feel overwhelmed figuring out where to begin. Or you may have been involved a good deal in helping others and noticed some ways you want to refine how you engage in social justice change efforts. I have found *Four Roles in Social Change: Helpers, Advocates, Organizers, and Rebels* by George Lakey (n.d.; with "thanks to social activist and strategist Bill Moyer") to be really helpful in reflecting on the strengths I have related to social justice change and also how to appreciate the efforts of others and refine my effectiveness when I seek to participate in social justice change efforts. Read through the following descriptions of the four roles, and see which resonate with your own style.

Helper—good at helping others in a respectful and affirmative manner; uses education, encouragement, and skill-sharing to foster empowerment and success.

Advocate—enjoys working with government organizations and other stakeholder organizations related to policy changes; uses coalitions and focuses on policy change for successful outcomes.

Organizer—works at a grassroots level and encourages leadership development by examining different points of view; uses both short-term and long-term visioning, planning, and training to ensure success.

Rebel—feels comfortable with direct actions, such as protests, using these actions to publicize institutional injustice in efforts to hold those in power accountable and bring about social justice change.

Although I have participated in each of these four roles, I am really drawn to the role of being an organizer. I feel like I am most effective in this role; more importantly, my resilience is increased by this role. I might engage in some of the other roles for time-limited activities, but I can always sense when my resilience starts going downhill because I feel overwhelmed and not able to focus.

In the next resilience practice, you'll explore these four life roles a little more.

RESILIENCE PRACTICE: The Four Roles in Social Change and Your Resilience Meter

Think of your overall amount of resilience—the reserve of energy you have to bounce back from difficult times as an LGBTQ person—and then think of that resilience energy as a meter. The resilience meter ticks up when you are engaged in social change efforts that increase your resilience, and ticks down when your resilience is decreased. Keep this in mind as you explore your aptitude for the four roles in social change and the likelihood of increasing your resilience when you engage in these roles:

Helper

What are your thoughts about the Helper role in relation to social change?

_____

_____

_____

What might be some drawbacks to the Helper role in relation to your resilience?

_____

_____

_____

Advocate

What are your thoughts about the Advocate role in relation to social change?

_____

_____

_____

What might be some drawbacks to the Advocate role in relation to your resilience?

_____

_____

_____

Organizer

What are your thoughts about the Organizer role in relation to social change?

_____

_____

_____

What might be some drawbacks to the Organizer role in relation to your resilience?

_____

_____

_____

Rebel

What are your thoughts about the Rebel role in relation to social change?

_____

_____

_____

What might be some drawbacks to the Rebel role in relation to your resilience?

_____

_____

_____

Now that you've reflected on these four roles, which were you drawn to the most—and the least? Are there any you feel pretty neutral about—like you could take it or leave it? Which roles did you rate highest and lowest? Were there overlaps for any role between the ratings you gave for your strengths and for the likelihood it would increase your resilience?

Targeting Your Involvement in Social Justice Change Efforts

With a clearer idea of what you like and don't like about the four roles and how they relate to your resilience, think about how you might want to not only get involved in social change efforts but also try out one of the four roles when anti-LGBTQ efforts are under way at the local, state, national, or international level. For instance, I work on social justice change related to issues of race/ethnicity, gender, and sexual orientation with LGBTQ people. I also work a lot outside of the LGBTQ community on certain issues, such as police brutality and mental health disability. In the next resilience practice, you can explore how you might want to engage in social justice change related to some of the common issues that specifically affect LGBTQ people. Again, it can be important to know how you might react in any one of these scenarios so you have an idea of what might increase or decrease your resilience.

RESILIENCE PRACTICE: Anticipating Your Resilience in Difficult Sociopolitical Times

In this resilience practice, you get to run through a few scenarios of anti-LGBTQ sociopolitics to see how you might need to anticipate effects on your resilience and build or protect it during these times. This is a quick check of how your resilience might be tested and what you might do in these situations to increase it. For each of the example scenarios, feel free to rephrase or expand to better fit you in terms of your multiple identities; for example, you might add considerations related to race/ethnicity, class, disability, and other salient identities. Remember that social change acts can range from small to sweeping and everything in between, and they include online change efforts like social media.

An anti-trans bathroom law is passed in your state.

What would you do related to social change that would increase your resilience?

_____

What other salient identities would affect you, your resilience, and your actions?

_____

An anti-LGBTQ rights ordinance is passed in your city.

What would you do related to social change that would increase your resilience?

_____

What other salient identities would affect you, your resilience, and your actions?

_____

Police have been targeting members of the LGBTQ community.

What would you do related to social change that would increase your resilience?

_____

What other salient identities would affect you, your resilience, and your actions?

_____

A judge denies LGBTQ partners the right to adopt a child.

What would you do related to social change that would increase your resilience?

_____

What other salient identities would affect you, your resilience, and your actions?

_____

An LGBTQ elder is abused in an assisted living center.

What would you do related to social change that would increase your resilience?

_____

What other salient identities would affect you, your resilience, and your actions?

_____

LGBTQ people are seeking asylum from a country with anti-LGBTQ policies.

What would you do related to social change that would increase your resilience?

_____

What other salient identities would affect you, your resilience, and your actions?

_____

This resilience practice assessed your feelings about potential involvement in social change at the local, state, national, and international levels related to anti-LGBTQ laws, policies, and practices. Often, anti-LGBTQ policies and practices can have even more severe impacts on people of color, people living with disabilities, and people with other marginalized identities. Although it is upsetting to think about the discrimination and inequities that exist in the world, you have the power to make change, in the form of your voice and your vision of how the world should be—and could be. And your vision of that world—influenced by your own life experiences—can be a great compass to use when anticipating how you might want to get involved in social change efforts.

Resilience Wrap-Up

This chapter was all about the resilience you can grow through helping others and giving back to your community. Keep the following in mind to make sure that helping and making social justice change increases your resilience and overall well-being:

- It's OK to feel however you feel about helping others. For some, it comes naturally and is a resilience booster; for others, it can feel draining.

- It's important to keep an eye on how much helping increases or decreases your resilience. People who love helping can overdo it, and people who think they do not like helping may actually be helping others in small but important ways that increase their resilience.

- Setting boundaries for your helping can help you stay on track as you grow your resilience. That nagging feeling that you are getting wiped out or overwhelmed can be a sign you've exceeded your helping capacity.

- There are many ways to effect community and social justice change, and you may fit into one or more of four roles: helper, advocate, organizer, and rebel.

- Each of the four roles calls on different strengths and challenges you to expand your comfort zone. Know your preferences and your dislikes related to these four roles and how your accompanying strengths and growing edges relate to your resilience.

- Knowing how you react—or might react—to anti-LGBTQ laws, policies, and practices can help you grow your resilience, because you are anticipating what you might need and how your multiple identities may play into your reactions and needs.

In Chapter 11, you'll pull together your learning from previous chapters to reflect on how you can keep growing and thriving as an LGBTQ person, as well as the needs and supports you have for this journey.

Growing and Thriving

Part of your resilience depends on learning to grow and thrive as a queer and/or trans person, and this chapter explores how practices of self-growth can move you in this direction. Self-growth includes spending time in self-reflection, as well as getting feedback from others you trust who support you in being the best possible *you*. Happily, through these efforts self-growth ultimately moves you toward greater thriving and resilience.

Love takes off masks that we fear we cannot live without and know we cannot live within.

—James Baldwin, Black, gay, cisgender,
author and activist

What Is Self-Growth?

"Self-growth" is one of those touchy-feely terms that can be hard to define. There are several definitions, but these generally agree that self-growth is a process of looking at your shortcomings or weaknesses (I prefer calling these growing edges) and identifying areas that you could strengthen.

You definitely know when self-growth is happening! You may feel a mixture of excitement, relief, motivation, and other positive emotions as you sense something important under way. When I learn something new about myself, I feel excited because it is an opportunity to be more aware of how this new learning plays out in my life. I also really appreciate learning new things about others and the world, because I think it helps me grow into a better person. That growth naturally strengthens my resilience. The more I can trust in my ability to grow and change, the more I can trust in my ability to bounce back when things are tough.

However, you might also feel some nervousness or pain related to self-growth, as in "Wow, I didn't know I had to grow in that direction." I felt this way the last time my partner said, "Hey, can you put the phone down and listen to me?" When she said this, honestly, I didn't feel a rush of "Yes, of course, sweetie!" I felt more, "Uh-oh, I messed up." Pretty soon afterward,

I used positive self-talk to ask myself how I could grow more in paying attention—and putting down my phone. And I felt really good about this direction in my self-growth. I had a feeling that growing my attention skills would be a benefit in all of my life, from my personal to my professional relationships—and it certainly has made a difference! I remember a time when I might have gotten more defensive about taking in this type of feedback. Now, I may have the initial emotional "oops" reaction, but I have shortened the time between when I notice this feeling and remember that feedback like this is an invitation to grow. And in any situation I get to decide whether I want to grow or not.

You can probably see that when you are queer and trans, self-growth is particularly tricky—but particularly important! You want and deserve to live an awesome life, and self-growth and feedback from others can help with that. However, because our community regularly receives anti-LGBTQ messages, it is crucial to know what kinds of messages from others feel good and right for you—and what kinds are designed to bring you down. In the following resilience practice, you'll explore your experiences of self-growth as an LGBTQ person.

RESILIENCE PRACTICE: Defining Your Own Self-Growth

In this resilience practice, reflect on the times in your life when you've experienced *positive* self-growth that helped (or continues to help) you affirm yourself as an LGBTQ person. Complete the following sentence stems:

I am growing the most as an LGBTQ person when

_____

_____

_____

I am growing the least as an LGBTQ person when

_____

_____

_____

The people who have supported me the most in my self-growth as an LGBTQ person have been

_____

_____

_____

The experiences or situations that have supported me the most in my self-growth as an LGBTQ person have been

_____

_____

_____

The obstacles I still face in my self-growth as an LGBTQ person are

_____

_____

_____

To support my self-growth as an LGBTQ person, I need

_____

_____

_____

As you completed this resilience practice, did any emotions come up? It can be natural to experience a range of emotions—sadness, frustration, happiness, fear—depending on your experiences of supportive people and situations in your life as an LGBTQ person. What insights did you have about the supports and obstacles for your self-growth as an LGBTQ person? Hold on to these insights as you read about making a regular practice of self-growth.

Making a Regular Practice of Self-Growth to Thrive

Your understanding of self-growth should be clearer now. You know when you are experiencing it—and you can have a variety of emotions as you grow and receive feedback. With a clearer understanding of what your own self-growth is, your resilience can increase as you set aside regular time for what helps you grow. Why set aside time for your self-growth? Well, it's a precious time that is just for you—not for anyone else. This may not seem that revolutionary, but the time you set aside for your own self-actualization (another term for self-growth) ticks your resilience meter up, and then you move into the thriving zone.

What is the thriving zone? Well, thriving means you are not just in a state of bouncing back from hard times. Thriving means you are flourishing and having feelings of success and prosperity. Thriving is not a state where you don't experience any adversity, but one in which the challenges you face (big and small) don't take you off course.

In my culture, we refer to thriving as following your purpose in life or your dharma. You don't have to be in pursuit of a spiritual or religious purpose, although you may be. Your purpose or dharma is the path you create for your life, with each step guided by your inner coach telling you how awesome you are and that you can trust yourself and your visions, goals, and dreams for your life. Sounds pretty cool, eh?

My dharma is certainly about helping others and being in the counseling profession, but during the time I was discovering who I was in terms of my gender, sexual orientation, and other identities, all my energy was devoted to simply surviving; even resilience took a backseat to my need to stay afloat and just make it through the day in school, college, and different work settings. Once I had LGBTQ mentors and people who modeled what my inner coach voice should look like (as you explored in Chapter 4), all of a sudden I had energy and support to reflect on my dharma. Then all the worries I had about not knowing what I should do with my life faded away. I realized not only that I had gifts, talents, and skills (as you explored in yourself earlier in this chapter), but that with these I could create a life path of honor, integrity, passion, and truth. Now, the dharma path can be hard work and require some discipline to follow, but it can also be super fun, as you can connect with similarly minded folks and community along the way. Read Seth Pardo's story of his resilience in finding and defining himself.

Just as with most things in my life, I thrive not because of what I did only for myself, but because of what so many others have done to pave the way for me and because of the support of so many loved ones. Growing up in Miami Beach in the early '80s was not particularly difficult. I lived a life of privilege, free from many forms of discrimination. I was, however, quite different from many of my peers, and I knew that very early. I knew that I wasn't like most of the other girls I knew—in fact, I was pretty certain I was unlike any of the other girls I knew. I never really came out to my parents as same-sex attracted; they figured it out, but it was never an issue. But when I came out to my parents as trans when I was fifteen, all of us looked at each other in silence for a while, not because of prejudice or judgment, but because nobody knew what to do next. My parents reminded me that they loved me no matter what, and that they weren't sure what was the best thing to do, but that we'd figure it out together. That day I came home from school exhausted from how it all started, and there were three books on my bed: Young, Gay and Proud [an anthology edited by Sasha Alyson and Lynne Yamaguchi Fletcher], Lou Sullivan's book on how to crossdress like an FTM transsexual [Information for the Female-to-Male Cross Dresser and Transsexual], *and a book about hormones and how they affect the body when someone pursues a medical transition from female to male. I think my mom had read them all before she gave them to me, which is good because up until that point, I don't think she had even considered what trans was. Many years later, we have more language with which to reflect on and talk about what was happening for me, and she said, "I'm sorry I didn't know what was happening for you." She commented on how hard things must have been and how awful she felt that she wasn't able to help me more then. I appreciated that very much, considering that she and I fought a great deal in my childhood and I just didn't have the language to explain why dresses made me feel so bad. My parents weren't the only sources of support. I had a core group of friends who accepted me for exactly who I was. In those days when trans identities didn't have the visibility they have today, we didn't have language to describe how I felt, but my core friends just got it that I should have been born male, and that was that. They treated me like one of the guys, they loved me like a boyfriend, and all of this contributed to my resilient growth and thriving as a trans person.*

In my later adulthood, when I was finally ready to begin my medical transition—once I was sure it wasn't just internalized homonegativity, or a rejection of just being female-bodied and attracted to women—I embraced therapy and developed a solid sense of self, grounded in self-love and appreciation for how hard it was growing up without having the language to talk about my frustration with gender and resentment for being so different. I learned through that self-exploration how to love my uniqueness and to celebrate my membership in community with other trans people.

—Seth Pardo, White, trans man, psychologist

Work through the following resilience practice to explore your dharma further as a way to increase both your resilience and your thriving. This resilience practice demonstrates how setting aside just a tiny amount of time to reflect on your self-growth and needs can increase your resilience and thriving.

RESILIENCE PRACTICE: Exploring How You Can Thrive as an LGBTQ Person

Think about your life without any constraints as an LGBTQ person. In this world of no restraints, what do you see yourself feeling, thinking, and doing? Respond to the following prompts from this point of view—experiencing complete freedom to manifest your visions, goals, and dreams for your life.

When I think of my purpose in life, I feel

_____

_____

_____

The visions, dreams, and goals for my life include

_____

_____

_____

If someone asked me about what my dharma—or purpose in life—is, I would say the following:

_____

_____

_____

As an LGBTQ person, my purpose in life has been influenced negatively by

_____

_____

_____

As an LGBTQ person, my purpose in life has been influenced positively by

_____

_____

_____

When I imagine realizing my visions, dreams, and goals for my life as an LGBTQ person,
I feel

_____

_____

_____

When I imagine bringing to life my visions, dreams, and goals as an LGBTQ person, these
additional identities matter to me:

_____

_____

_____

How do you feel after making a little time for your own self-growth and reflection on your
dharma? As you wrote about your purpose, was it easy, hard, or somewhere in between? When
you explored your purpose in life as an LGBTQ person, did responding feel simple or more
difficult? There are no wrong responses, of course, in this or any other resilience practice. And
it's certainly understandable, if you haven't thought about your dharma before as an LGBTQ
person, that you felt a bit stressed as you completed your responses. With this activity, there is
good stress ("Oh wow—I am exploring something that I don't yet know about myself!") and
bad stress ("Oh no—I should already know this about myself!")—and you are going for the
good stress that can accompany the excitement of learning something new about yourself. It is
important, however, to consider how your answers might change if you were to respond again
in a week, month, or year. (If you'd like to complete this resilience practice again, you can
download the worksheet that's available at http://www.newharbinger.com/39461.) Making it a
regular practice to come back to explore your visions, dreams, and goals for your life will help
you increase your resilience and your thriving.

Hopefully life is long. Do stuff you will enjoy thinking about and telling stories about for many years to come.

—Rachel Maddow, White, lesbian, cisgender, media person

Practicing Self-Love to Thrive

In Chapter 4, you explored self-worth and self-esteem, two important components of resilience. Self-love takes that valuing of yourself even deeper. I have a friend who describes it as falling in love with *you*. Self-love is a deep practice of thriving as an LGBTQ person that can help you identify the steps on your thriving dharma path. Self-love is like all the individual parts of the resilience wheel you have learned about so far in this workbook, rolled up together in one big ball of unconditional positive regard for yourself. Here are some of my own favorite self-love activities:

- Taking time to walk outside during the day

- Making time to go hear live music

- Taking long baths and listening to music

- Practicing yoga and meditation each day

- Saying affirmations out loud

- Paying attention to when I need to rest

- Taking naps!

- Challenging the negative gremlin critic in my head

- Traveling and going on new adventures

- Hiking among really tall trees in the mountains

This is just a sample of my self-love practices. They feel really good to do! I hope they may remind you of your own favorite things that bring you into the present moment and make you feel cared for by yourself. Although you feel good when you practice self-love, it can also be complicated. Depending on how much anti-LGBTQ experience you've had—or are currently experiencing—it can feel like you don't have time to practice self-love, even though self-love can be a balm for the soul and help you get through those tough times. It can be hard to remember to do self-love when you are facing a lot of pressures, distractions, or expectations as an LGBTQ person. But, like self-growth, you can learn to love yourself through personal practice, support, and self-reflection. Do the next resilience practice to further explore the possibilities for self-love.

///

RESILIENCE PRACTICE: Practicing Self-Love with Depth and Intention

In this resilience practice, you'll reflect on self-love practices that entail self-care, mindfulness, and other ways to feel safe and whole as an LGBTQ person.

What are some of the self-love practices you currently do for yourself?

_____

_____

_____

What are some self-love practices you would like to have more of in your life?

_____

_____

_____

What everyday self-love practices could you add?

_____

_____

_____

What are the barriers to integrating these self-love practices into your everyday life?

_____

_____

_____

Name three brief, doable everyday self-love practices to integrate into your life now.

_____

_____

_____

Name three people you can talk with to keep you accountable for these three everyday self-love practices.

_____

_____

_____

Did you notice there are some self-love practices you already do for yourself? Did you list a lot of self-love practices? Even five minutes a day of being more sweet, kind, and loving to yourself can make a big difference! If it was hard for you to identify any self-love practices, be gentle with yourself and start conversations with others you trust about how they integrate self-love practices into their everyday lives.

Getting Your Resilience Wheel Turning toward Thriving

Now that you are nearing the end of this workbook, it is time to reflect on your overall resilience by taking a look back at what you have explored before. Taking a moment to review all the components of your resilience as an LGBTQ person will help you stay on track in building your resilience through each spoke in the resilience wheel.

It's pretty cool to look at the resilience wheel again and realize that these spokes are concepts that you can put into action right now. In the introduction, you probably saw the resilience wheel as just a figure based on research findings and best practices. But now that you have personally explored each component of the resilience wheel, isn't it great to realize that you have made it *yours*?

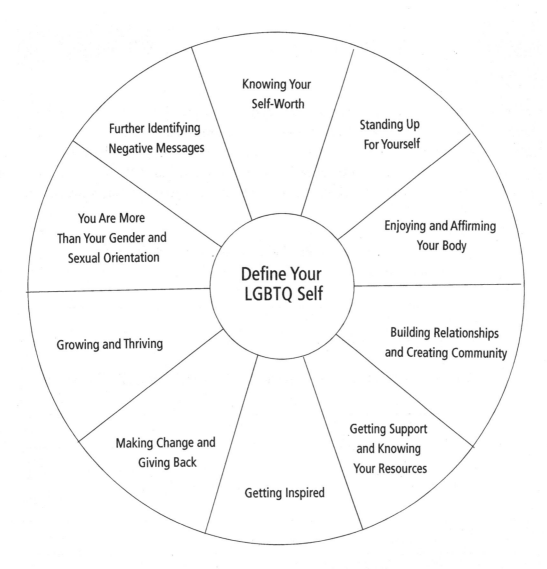

Each of us has our own version of the resilience wheel. Your resilience wheel is unique to you. Your resilience wheel celebrates your uniqueness as an LGBTQ person. Your resilience wheel highlights the important support and needs you have as a queer or trans person. Your resilience wheel reminds you of your self-worth, and the importance of having supportive resources and standing up for yourself when you experience discrimination. Your resilience wheel encourages you to love yourself—your body, mind, and spirit. And along the way to growing your resilience wheel, you get to be inspired and make change within yourself and the world in ways that feel right to you, to give back to others. Most importantly, the components of your own resilience wheel keep you mindful that you can do more than just survive in this world. Your dharma as an LGBTQ person is to thrive. Period. Do this final resilience practice to reflect on the different elements of your resilience wheel and how to continually strengthen it.

RESILIENCE PRACTICE: Putting Your Resilience Wheel into Action

As you respond to this resilience practice, you may want to turn back to earlier chapters in this workbook. On the left, rate each component of your resilience wheel on a scale of 1 to 5 (1 being the lowest and 5 being the highest) in terms of your current understanding of the concepts and integrating a resilience spoke into your everyday life. After rating a resilience spoke, write down any thoughts you have right now about how to grow your resilience in this area:

_____   Getting Real: Defining Your LGBTQ Self in a World That Demands Conformity (Chapter 1)

_____

_____

_____   You Are More Than Your Gender and Sexual Orientation (Chapter 2)

_____

_____

_____   Further Identifying Negative Messages (Chapter 3)

_____

_____

_____   Knowing Your Self-Worth (Chapter 4)

_____

_____

_____   Standing Up for Yourself (Chapter 5)

_____

_____

_____ Affirming and Enjoying Your Body (Chapter 6)

_____

_____

_____ Building Relationships and Creating Community (Chapter 7)

_____

_____

_____ Getting Support and Knowing Your Resources (Chapter 8)

_____

_____

_____ Getting Inspired (Chapter 9)

_____

_____

_____ Making Change and Giving Back (Chapter 10)

_____

_____

_____ Growing and Thriving (this chapter)

_____

_____

How did you feel running through the different components of your resilience wheel? What were the areas you rated higher or lower? Did you notice any themes related to these ratings? It can be helpful to have someone you trust to talk with about your resilience wheel whenever you need to. The most important person who checks in with your resilience wheel, of course, is you. You are in charge of your life as an LGBTQ person, even when life tries to tell you otherwise. Your resilience reminds you of your inherent right to thrive as a queer or trans person on this planet.

Resilience Wrap-Up

As this workbook closes, I hope that you not only have learned something about resilience, but also have made a deep commitment to yourself to be kind, gentle, compassionate, and loving. For queer and trans people, there is so much in the world that we think and feel is out of our control. And when it comes to queer and trans oppression and discrimination, there's so much you actually can't control. You can, however, promise yourself you'll never take yourself down in the way that it seems the world wants to. That doesn't mean simply being strong, nor just learning how to take things in stride, nor ignoring discrimination. In this workbook, you have learned that intentionally developing each component of your resilience—even one at a time—builds something no one can ever take away from you, no matter what your circumstances are: the recognition and appreciation of your inherent worth as a queer or trans person. My wish for you is to not only remember your own unique beauty and resilience as an LGBTQ person, but also to remind others in our community to shine their lights proudly into this world.

Acknowledgments

There are numerous people I would like to thank for their support in developing this text. First, to the many people I have worked with in studying queer and trans resilience—friends, community members and collaborators, research participants, colleagues, and students—I am eternally thankful and more resilient as a result of each of you!

I have immensely enjoyed working with the amazing folks on the editorial team at New Harbinger. Ryan Buresh, you have been a true gem to work with, from book inception to publication. I have appreciated everything you have done to support me as an author and for your impeccable communication along the way. You are incredibly trustworthy and also a fierce advocate for authors. Thank you! To the top-notch reviewers at New Harbinger—Clancy Drake and Erin Raber, who gave me helpful and timely feedback—wow! The book is so much stronger as a result of your keen attention to the content and my overall goals for this workbook. Thanks as well to Vicraj Gill for preparing the online content so that people can access some of the resilience practices from this text; to Amy Shoup for designing the book cover; and to Kristi Hein for final copyediting, good humor, and encouragement. I am incredibly grateful for my dear friend and brother, Priyanka Sinha, who designed and revised the Queer and Trans Resilience Wheel figure. Thank you for believing in this book and the Trans Resilience Project.

And to the readers of this workbook: however you have come to pick up this workbook or read it online, it is my greatest hope that you become your most resilient and thriving self while reading it. I also hope you will pass it on to those who may need it most. My favorite author—Arundhati Roy—said it the best: "Another world is not only possible, she is on her way. On a quiet day, I can hear her breathing." *You* are that possible world.

Resources

Books

Beyond Magenta: Transgender Teens Speak Out by Susan Kulkin (Walker Books, 2016)

The Gender Quest Workbook: A Guide for Teens and Young Adults Exploring Gender Identity by Rylan Jay Testa, Deborah Coolhart, and Jayme Peta (Instant Help, 2015)

Lost Prophet: The Life and Times of Bayard Rustin by John D'Emilio (University of Chicago Press, 2004)

Mindfulness and Acceptance for Gender and Sexual Minorities by Matthew Skinta, Aisling Curtin, and John Pachankis (New Harbinger, 2016)

A Queer History of the United States by Michael Bronski (Beacon Press, 2012)

Sister Outsider by Audre Lorde (Crossing Press, 2007)

The Velvet Rage: Overcoming the Pain of Growing Up in a Straight Man's World by Alan Downs (HighBridge, 2012)

Websites

Audre Lorde Project
   www.alp.org

Gender Spectrum
   www.genderspectrum.org

GLSEN
   www.glsen.org

GSA Network
   www.gsanetwork.org

Lambda Legal

www.lambdalegal.org

National Center for Transgender Equality

www.ncte.org

PFLAG

www.pflag.org

Safe Schools Coalition

www.safeschoolscoalition.org

SAGE

www.sageusa.org

The Trevor Project

www.thetrevorproject.org

References

Institute of Medicine. (2011). *The health of lesbian, gay, bisexual, and transgender people: Building a foundation for better understanding.* Washington, DC: National Academy of Sciences.

Kosciw, J. G., Greytak, E. A., Giga, N. M., Villenas, C., & Danischewski, D. J. (2017). The 2015 National School Climate Survey: The experiences of lesbian, gay, bisexual, transgender, and queer youth in our nation's schools. New York, NY: GLSEN.

Lakey, G. (n.d.). Four roles in social change: Helpers, advocates, organizers, and rebels. Retrieved from http://www.newjimcroworganizing.org/tools.html.

Masten, A. S. (2015). *Ordinary magic: Resilience in development.* New York, NY: Guilford Press.

Meyer, I. H. (2003). Prejudice, social stress, and mental health in lesbian, gay and bisexual populations: Conceptual issues and research evidence. *Psychological Bulletin, 129,* 674–697. doi:10.1037/0033–2909.129.5.674.

———. (2015). Resilience in the study of minority stress and health of sexual and gender minorities. *Psychology of Sexual Orientation and Gender Diversity, 2*(3), 209–213. doi:10.1037/sgd0000132.

Rosenberg, M. (1965). *Society and the adolescent self-image.* Princeton, NJ: Princeton University Press.

Russell, S. T., Ryan, C., Toomey, R. B., Diaz, R. M., & Sanchez, J. (2011). Lesbian, gay, bisexual, and transgender adolescent school victimization: Implications for young adult health and adjustment. *Journal of School Health, 81*(5), 223–230. doi:10.1111/j.1746–1561.2011.00583.x

Singh, A. A., Hays, D. G., & Watson, L. (2011). Strategies in the face of adversity: Resilience strategies of transgender individuals. *Journal of Counseling and Development, 89*(1), 20–27. doi:10.1002/j.1556–6678.2011.tb00057.x.

Singh, A. A., & McKleroy, V. S. (2011). "Just getting out of bed is a revolutionary act": The resilience of transgender people of color who have survived traumatic life events. *International Journal of Traumatology, 17*(2), 34–44. doi: 10.1177/1534765610369261.

Singh, A. A. (March 2012). Transgender youth of color and resilience: Negotiating oppression, finding support. *Sex Roles: A Journal of Research*, 1–13. doi:10.1007/s1199–012–0149-z.

Singh, A. A., Meng, S., & Hansen, A. (2014). "I am my own gender:" Resilience strategies of trans youth. *Journal of Counseling & Development*, 92(2), 208–218. doi:10.1002/j.1556–6676.2014.00150.x.

Sue, D. W. S., & Sue, D. S. (2015). *Counseling the culturally diverse: Theory and practice* (7th ed.). New York, NY: Wiley.

Anneliese Singh, PhD, LPC, is associate dean of diversity, equity, and inclusion in the College of Education at the University of Georgia, and professor in the department of counseling and human development services. She is cofounder of the Georgia Safe Schools Coalition, an intersectional organization; and founder of the Trans Resilience Project. She resides in Avondale Estates, GA.

Foreword writer **Diane Ehrensaft, PhD**, is a developmental and clinical psychologist in the San Francisco Bay Area. She is director of mental health and founding member of the Child and Adolescent Gender Center—a partnership between the University of California, San Francisco, and community agencies to provide comprehensive interdisciplinary services and advocacy to gender non-conforming/transgender children and youth, and their families.

MORE BOOKS *from*
NEW HARBINGER PUBLICATIONS

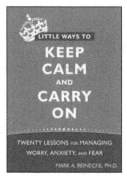

**LITTLE WAYS TO
KEEP CALM & CARRY ON**

Twenty Lessons for
Managing Worry, Anxiety & Fear

978-1572248816 / US $15.95

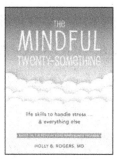

**THE MINDFUL
TWENTY-SOMETHING**

Life Skills to Handle Stress...
& Everything Else

978-1626254893 / US $16.95

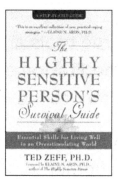

**THE HIGHLY SENSITIVE
PERSON'S SURVIVAL GUIDE**

Essential Skills for Living Well in
an Overstimulating World

978-1572243965 / US $18.95

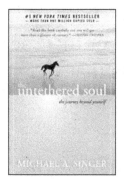

THE UNTETHERED SOUL

The Journey Beyond Yourself

978-1572245372 / US $16.95

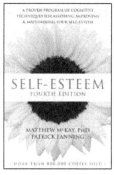

**SELF-ESTEEM,
FOURTH EDITION**

A Proven Program of Cognitive
Techniques for Assessing, Improving
& Maintaining Your Self-Esteem

978-1626253933 / US $17.95

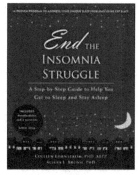

**END THE INSOMNIA
STRUGGLE**

A Step-by-Step Guide to Help You
Get to Sleep & Stay Asleep

978-1626253438 / US $24.95

new harbinger publications
1-800-748-6273 / newharbinger.com

(VISA, MC, AMEX / prices subject to change without notice)

Follow Us

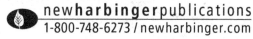

Don't miss out on new books in the subjects that interest you.
Sign up for our **Book Alerts** at **newharbinger.com/bookalerts**

Did you know there are **free tools** you can download for this book?

Free tools are things like **worksheets**, **guided meditation exercises**, and **more** that will help you get the most out of your book.

You can download free tools for this book—whether you bought or borrowed it, in any format, from any source—from the New Harbinger website. All you need is a NewHarbinger.com account. Just use the URL provided in this book to view the free tools that are available for it. Then, click on the "download" button for the free tool you want, and follow the prompts that appear to log in to your NewHarbinger.com account and download the material.

You can also save the free tools for this book to your **Free Tools Library** so you can access them again anytime, just by logging in to your account! Just look for this button on the book's free tools page. ➤

+ Save this to my free tools library

If you need help accessing or downloading free tools, visit **newharbinger.com/faq** or contact us at **customerservice@newharbinger.com**.